THE EASY KETO CHAFFLE COOKBOOK

Sweet and Savory Ketogenic Recipes to Boost Your Metabolism and Increase Fat Burning. Low-Carb Chaffles to Achieve Your Diet Goals and Start a Healthier Life

Tasty Food Academy

KETO CHAFFLE
6 AWESOME ways!

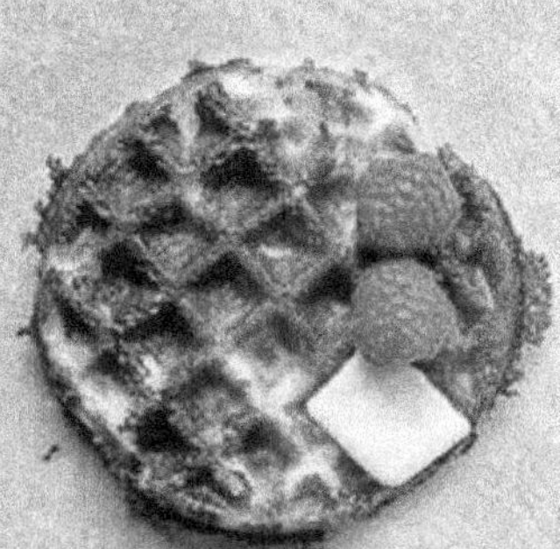

traditional
1/2 cup mozzarella, 1 egg
+ 1 tablespoon almond flour

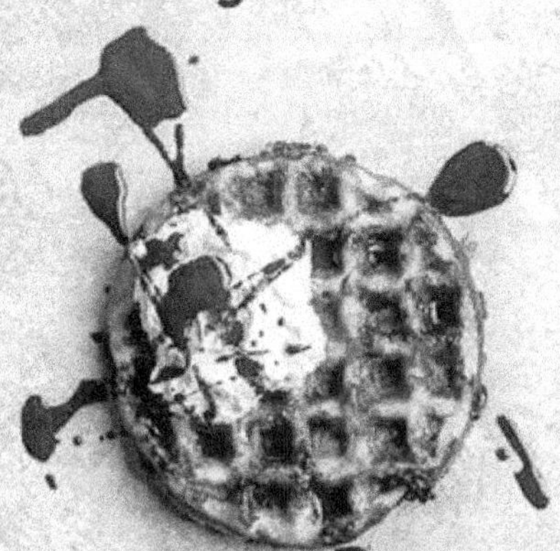

chocolate chip
1 tablespoon erythritol, 1/2 teaspoon vanilla
2 tablespoons chocolate chips

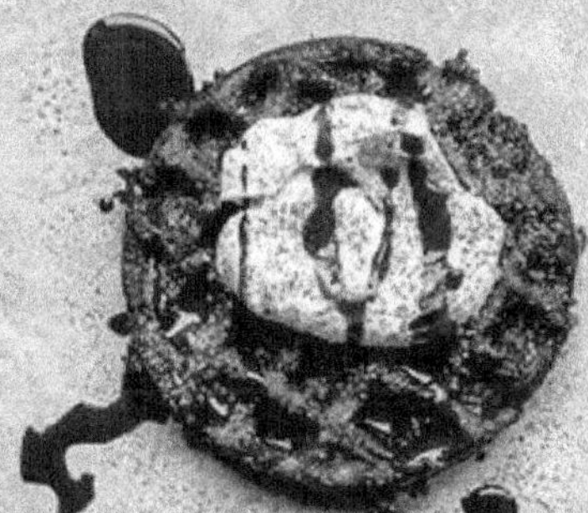

brownie
1 tablespoon erythritol, 2 tablespoons chocolate chips
2 tablespoons cocoa powder, 1/2 teaspoon vanilla
+ 1 tablespoon cream cheese

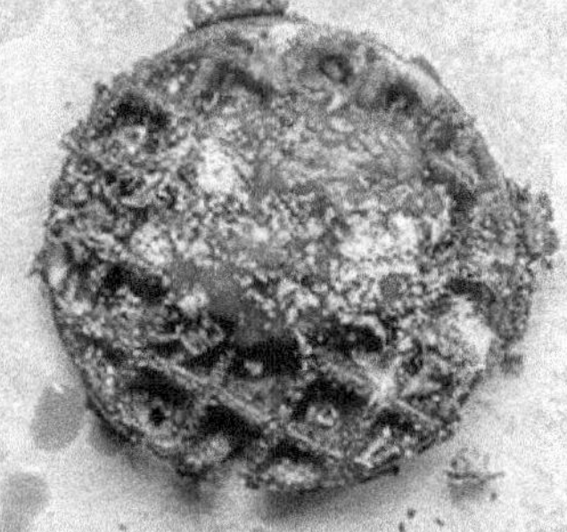

pizza
1 teaspoon italian seasoning
+ 1/4 cup pepperoni

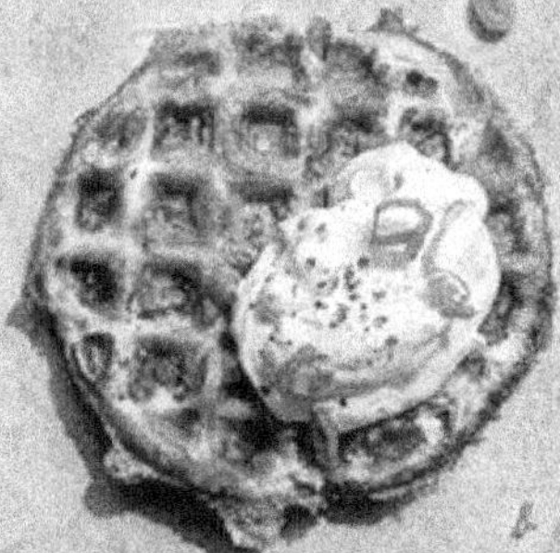

ham + cheese
1/4 cup ham + 1/4 cup green onions

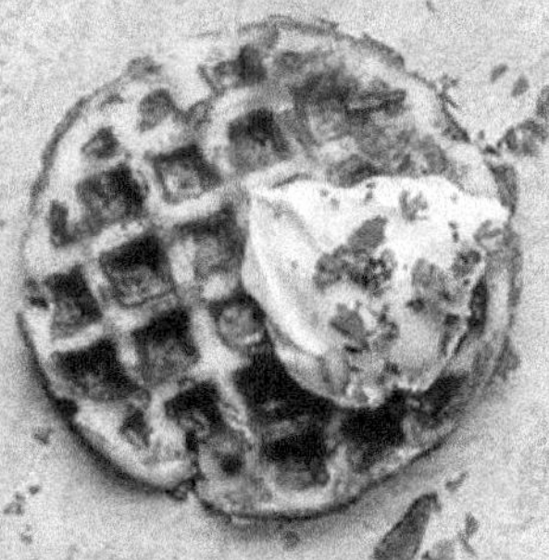

jalapeno popper
2 tablespoons cream cheese, 1 tablespoon jalapeno
2 tablespoons bacon

DISCLAIMER

The publisher and authors of this book show and teach you techniques of cooking and fixing foods; however, this book is independently published and is not affiliated with, sponsored by, or endorsed or affiliated with, or by any of the products mentioned in this book. All other company and product names are the Trademarks™ of their respective owners. The author reserves the right to make any changes he/she deems necessary to future versions of the publication to ensure its accuracy.

Special Notes for the Recipes in this Book:

The recipes in this book may include raw eggs. Raw eggs may contain bacteria. It is recommended that you purchase certified salmonella-free eggs from a reliable source and store them in the refrigerator. You should not feed raw eggs to babies or small kids. Likewise, pregnant women, elderly persons, or those with a compromised immune system should not eat raw eggs.

This book may also contain peanuts in some of the recipes. Please consult your physician if you have allergies to any particular foods before cooking these recipes. Neither the author nor the publisher claims responsibility for adverse effects resulting from the use of the recipes and/or information found within this book.

The information contained in this book is for entertainment purposes only. The author does not assume any liability whatsoever for the use of or inability to use any or all information contained in this book and accepts no responsibility for any loss or damages of any kind that may be incurred by the reader as a result of actions arising from the use of the information in this book. The content represents the opinion of the author and is based on the author's personal experience and observations.

Use this information at your own risk.

No part of this book may be reproduced or transmitted in any form or by any means, electronic or mechanical, including photocopying, recording, or by any information storage or retrieval system, without express written permission from the author, except in the case of brief quotations embodied in critical articles and reviews – or except by a reviewer who may quote brief passages in a review.

TABLE OF CONTENTS

Conclusion **414**

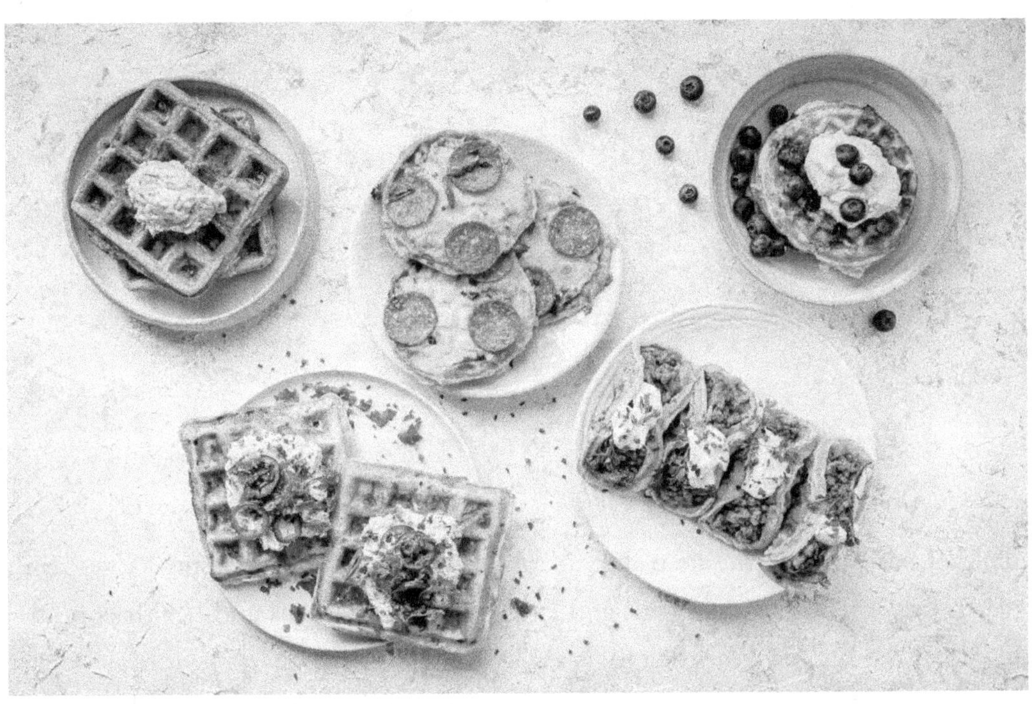

INTRODUCTION

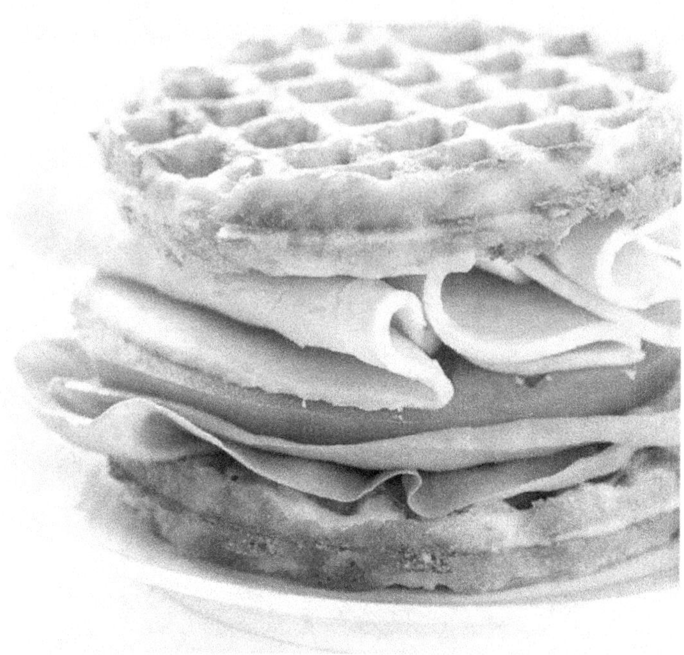

The Ketogenic diet, also named the keto diet, is a high-fat—moderate protein—low-carb approach to eating. The diet is used as both a treatment and cure for some diseases and health conditions. The diet became popular over the last few years due to its ability to help with weight loss, energy levels, and overall health. Basically, the idea behind the diet is to cover all three macronutrients. When following a Ketogenic diet, you are expected to consume a minimum of 60% of your calories each day from fat in order to stay in ketosis. In addition, you are also encouraged to eat as much protein as you can from sources such as meats, dairy, and even non-dairy sources like nuts and seeds.

In the low-carb world, the word **'Chaffle'** appeared and took social media by storm. Suddenly, every keto diet follower got astonished by the idea of using two special ingredients that have few carbohydrates but rich in proteins, fats, and other essential vitamins and minerals. The waffle maker became the need of every keto kitchen, and individuals following the Ketogenic diet found their new love.

This new addition to the keto diet is not only healthy, but the possibilities to experiment with new recipes are countless. Furthermore, it has also made it easy for keto followers to follow their diet and controlling their cravings for flour-based foods.

In simple words, chaffles are low-carb waffles—they are called chaffle because cheese is used as their base ingredient. Cheese and waffle by combining these words, you will get delicious chaffles.

The benefits of Ketogenic chaffles are that they are completely customizable and nutritious.

Keto Chaffles is a perfect recipe to try keto. They are made using coconut flour, egg whites, and cream cheese. They come in the form of pancakes and waffles. You can also make it into muffins or pieces of bread.

You can make your Keto Chaffles any way you want them to be, whether it is as pancakes, waffles, or muffins. You can add various ingredients and toppings to give them more flavors. It is important not to let the chaffles dry out while they are cooking, so be a little creative. There are many ways to top your keto chaffles, like bacon, creamy cheese, strawberry, or peach. You can also put other flavors like coffee, vanilla, or chocolate sauces if you want.

There are many benefits to enjoying keto chaffles. They have a high number of protein and fiber, which is a great combination to help with energy levels and feeling full while eating keto. On top of this, they have no carbs at all and are very low in sugar, so they will not affect blood glucose levels. Keto chaffles also contain healthy fats that make them a great choice for those following a low-carb or Ketogenic diet.

Another great thing about the keto chaffle is that it is super low in calories and carbs. Keto chaffles only have around 16 g of carbohydrates per serving. At the same time, each serving may contain only around 170 calories.

Keto eats fewer carbs, and it has truly gone ahead solid in the preceding eighteen months. It's an incredible method to shed those undesirable pounds fast, yet additionally, an extraordinary method to get slim and remain as such. Those who have tried the Keto Diet are still on it; it's something beyond an eating routine. It's a lifestyle, a totally new lifestyle. Nevertheless, similar to any significant shift in our lives, it's anything but a simple one; it takes a mind-boggling measure of responsibility and assurance.

Although there may be transitional pains as your body adapts to a new way of eating, these are short-lived, and the long-term benefits far outweigh them. There have been several surveys completed which indicate a keto diet can assist with preventing serious illnesses, such as cancer and Alzheimer's. Perhaps, more importantly, is the increased levels of energy you will have once you commit to the keto diet. Your body will become familiarized with burning fat and will happily continue to do so as there is always a plentiful supply of fat!

In addition to the inspiration provided here, there are many forums online which will offer support and advice as you travel along the keto diet journey. Indeed, you will soon be eager to share your own experiences and make improvements to these recipes to suit your own tastes!

Chapter 1.

KETOGENIC DIET

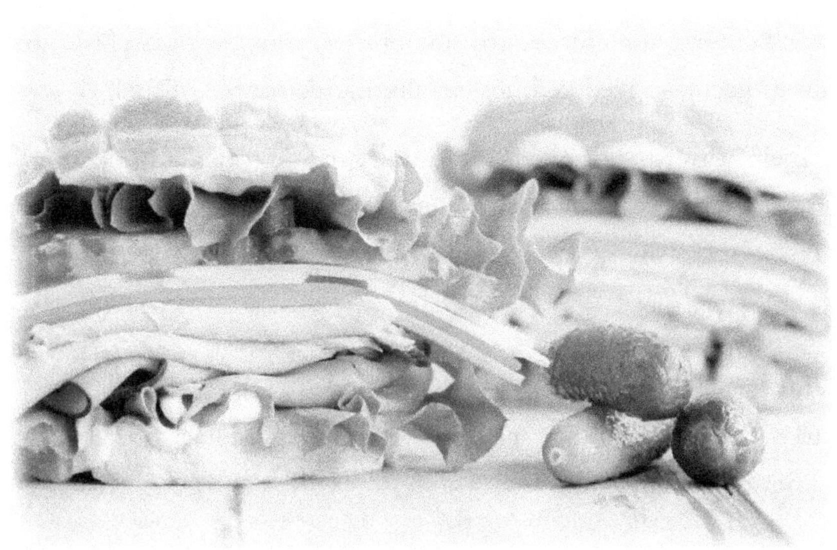

KETO DIET EXPLAINED

Keto diet is short for "Ketogenic." This is a high-fat content diet which purpose is to turn your body into a true fat-burning machine.

The way the keto diet achieves that is by changing the way your body converts food into energy. Usually, your body takes energy from carbohydrates by turning them into glucose. When you eat very few carbs and a lot of fat, it puts you in ketosis.

AND WHAT IS KETOSIS?

The term ketosis relates to a by-product of breaking down fat into useable energy, called ketones.

This fat can be derived from fat stores of the body or directly from a diet. Ketosis is caused by diet is referred to as "nutritional ketosis." Ketones are used by the body to power itself directly.

This process of breaking down fat into useful energy is similar to the process that carbohydrates undergo when turned into glucose to fuel the body. In other words, glucose is to carbohydrates what ketones are too fat.

What Are Ketones?

When your body doesn't get enough glucose from your diet, your liver starts to turn your body's fat and fat from your diet into molecules called ketones, an alternative source of fuel.

The keto diet is the main way to get your body running on ketones. Other ways include intermittent fasting, taking certain keto supplements, and using up your glucose reserves by exercising.

Ketogenic Health Benefits

- **Burns body fat**

Once you're on a keto diet, your body uses fat from your diet as well as stored body fat for energy. This helps people stay at a healthy weight.

- **Reduces appetite**

Ketones can suppress ghrelin—your hunger hormone—and increase cholecystokinin (CCK), which makes you feel full. Reduced appetite makes it easier to go without eating for longer periods, which encourages your body to remedy its fat stores for energy.

- **Reduces inflammation**

Inflammation is your body's natural reaction to an invader it considers harmful. But too much inflammation raises your risk of health and digestion problems. A keto diet is able to reduce inflammation in the body by switching off the inflammatory mechanisms and producing fewer free radicals.

- **Fuels your brain**

Ketones can offer a good portion of your brain's energy needs, more than the energy you get from glucose. The brain consists of more than 60% fat. That means it highly needs fat to work as it should, and the quality fats you eat on a Ketogenic diet are ideal for feeding the brain.

- **Increases energy**

When your body uses ketones for fuel, the same energy slumps as when you're eating a lot of carbs don't happen. Your body can easily tap into its fat stores for energy when your metabolism is in fat-burning mode. That means no more energy slumps or brain fog. Ketosis also helps to create more mitochondria, the power generators in your cells. Having more energy in your cells results in more energy to get stuff done.

- **Curb's cravings**

Fat is a satiating macronutrient. You eat more smart fats on keto, you feel fuller, longer.

Grasping the Ketogenic Diet

For people who have never tried the Ketogenic Diet, it can be a daunting task for many. Regardless of your goals or how long you've been on a diet, our cookbook has the information you need. For its main goal is to help you reach your weight loss or fat loss goals.

The Ketogenic Diet is a low carbohydrate, moderate protein, and high-fat diet. This lifestyle change provides you with an amazing amount of flexibility in achieving your goals. You'll be able to create a healthy eating plan that is tailored specifically for your needs and goals.

How to Blend Meals on the Keto Diet

The Keto diet is a great way to lose weight without starving. However, it's always helpful to know how people with the Keto diet cook their meals.

The Keto diet is based on low-carb, high-protein meals that are high in fat. This type of diet restricts your intake of carbs, which means most vegetables and fruits don't make the cut. If you eat a lot of carbohydrates like fruits, grains, and beans, you'll definitely miss out on all of the healthy benefits. However, there are plenty of different ways to make delicious meals without meat and dairy products.

You can add meat or cheese to many recipes and that would be considered keto-friendly without adding too much volume or carb content. For example, meals like "Zucchini Pizza Crust" or "Salmon with Black Bean Salsa" are both keto-friendly thanks to their high-fat content. Furthermore, your recipes can also be modified to include low-carb ingredients like almond flour or coconut flour.

Even if you want to lose weight or just change up your favorite recipes, the Keto diet has something for everyone! The greatest part is that there are no restrictions when it comes to what you can eat on this diet. Whether you want sweet or savory foods, there are plenty of options available to suit your personal tastes and eating preferences.

Chapter 2.

WHAT ARE THE ADVANTAGES OF KETOSIS?

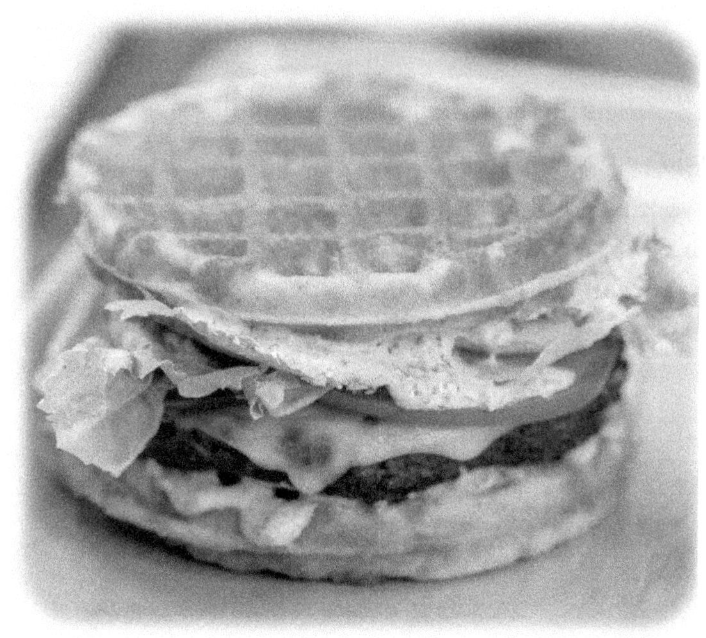

CORRELATION BETWEEN CALORIES AND KETOSIS

Have you ever heard not to count calories on the keto diet?

I'll explain it.

Calories are the amounts of energy present in your food, which means the amounts of energy that you derive from the foods that you eat. Fats, proteins, and carbs contribute to the calorie build in the body with different levels of contribution. For example:

- 1 g carbohydrate = 4 calories = 4 units of energy
- 1 g protein = 4 calories = 4 units of energy
- 1 g fat = 9 calories = 9 units of energy

Throughout the day, the body uses energy for smooth running. Averagely, adults burn between 1800 and 2600 calories per day, which will either be sourced from the foods eaten or from your fat stores.

28

Now, how does this affect ketosis?

While the different macronutrients contribute to calorie build in the body, their usage style will differ. Some foods burn extra calories better than others. For example, your body will need to work extra hard to break down protein than it will for carbohydrates. On the other hand, it will be faster for fats.

On the keto diet, the goal is to increase the number of calories sourced from fats rather than carbs to keep you in ketosis. Hence, a healthy boosting of calories through fats on the keto diet is sure to keep your ketosis.

CODEPENDENT BY FATS, PROTEINS, AND CARBOHYDRATES

I have heard many keto dieters condemn carbohydrates as if they were some dreadful ingredients. Not so! Equally like fats, proteins, and other micronutrients, carbs play an essential role in our bodies. Hence, understanding how they work with other nutrients is vital instead of condemnation.

Carbohydrates are an energy-fueling unit that the brain relies on for functioning. On a regular high-carb diet, carb reserves called glycogen serve as the primary source of energy to the brain and other organs in the body. However, these glycogen walls break down further into sucrose (sugars), which in excess may lead to high blood sugar; hence, varying related ailments caused. On the other hand, science proves that carbohydrates tend to be an inconsistent energy-fueling unit to the brain. This effect prevents the brain from functioning steadily and, therefore, the need for more carb intake to keep up with smooth work.

After much research to curb this problem, the keto diet was formulated. While the body falls back on carbs to provide energy when in excess, fats were realized to be an alternative and more sustainable fueling unit. By feeding on more fats and fewer carbs, the body is restructured to source its energy from fat stores found in the liver known as ketones—a water-soluble molecule produced from fatty acids.

Hence, the keto diet's goal is to push the body to provide more ketones than glycogen, which implies the dietary ratio stated earlier.

Meanwhile, how do proteins play in? Although we focus on fats in this case, the body must still feed on a balanced diet with the necessary nutrients playing in. Proteins are very crucial for growth, and so, a monitored amount in every meal must be included. Proteins break down into amino acids, which will often aid with muscle, bone, skin, nails, and cartilage building. However, an excess intake on the keto diet will quickly drive you out of ketosis as amino acids eventually increase the amount of insulin in the body.

In the keto diet, you have to consume healthy fats that can fulfill the needs of the carbohydrates in your body. For this purpose, one has to consume healthy fats and proteins. We all know chaffle is made up of healthy cheese and sugar-free ingredients. Cheese is undoubtedly a great source of fats, and this is the main reason that makes chaffle an excellent breakfast item for those on a low-carb diet.

Chapter 3.
WHAT IS A KETO CHAFFLE?

TYPES OF KETO CHAFFLES

Some of the usual ingredients you will use for a sweet chaffle are mozzarella cheese, milk, cocoa, cinnamon, almond flour, and low-carb sweeteners such as swerve or allulose. Mozzarella can be used in savory chaffles, but stronger, saltier cheeses such as cheddar or Colby jack are often combined with ingredients such as garlic powder, all bagel seasoning, tomato, jalapenos, etc.

CHAFFLE VARIATIONS

- **Plain.** Chaffles are incredible, all alone as a morning meal nourishment. You can serve them up close by bacon, eggs, avocado, and other standard keto breakfast charge.
- **Keto chaffle sandwich.** Create two chaffles and use them as bread for your preferred sandwich.
- **Chaffle dessert.** Attempt one of the sweet chaffle varieties recorded beneath and present with keto maple syrup or your most loved keto frozen yogurt.
- **Sweet chaffles:** Sprinkle cinnamon, vanilla extract, and low carb sweetener of your choice.
- **Pumpkin chaffles:** Drizzle pumpkin pie spice, maple extract, and low carb sweetener
- **Chocolate chaffles:** Sprinkle cacao powder or unsweetened cocoa powder, vanilla extract, low carb sweetener, and sugar-free chocolate chips.
- **Peanut butter chaffles:** Add peanut butter, vanilla extract, low carb sweetener, and top with chopped peanuts and a drizzle of peanut butter
- **Almond butter chaffles:** Add almond butter, vanilla extract, low carb sweetener, and top with strawberries, raspberries, blueberries, and a drizzle of almond butter.

FOR SAVORY CHAFFLES

- **2-Ingredient chaffles:** The original chaffle recipe uses ½ cup mozzarella cheese and 1 large egg.
- **Pizza chaffles:** Cook chaffle batter until crispy, then top with marinara sauce, shredded mozzarella, pepperoni, cherry tomatoes, and basil.
- **Chaffle sandwiches:** Cook the batter until crispy, then stuff with any ingredients you prefer.

You can alter your chaffle in a wide range of ways. Here are a couple of alternatives.

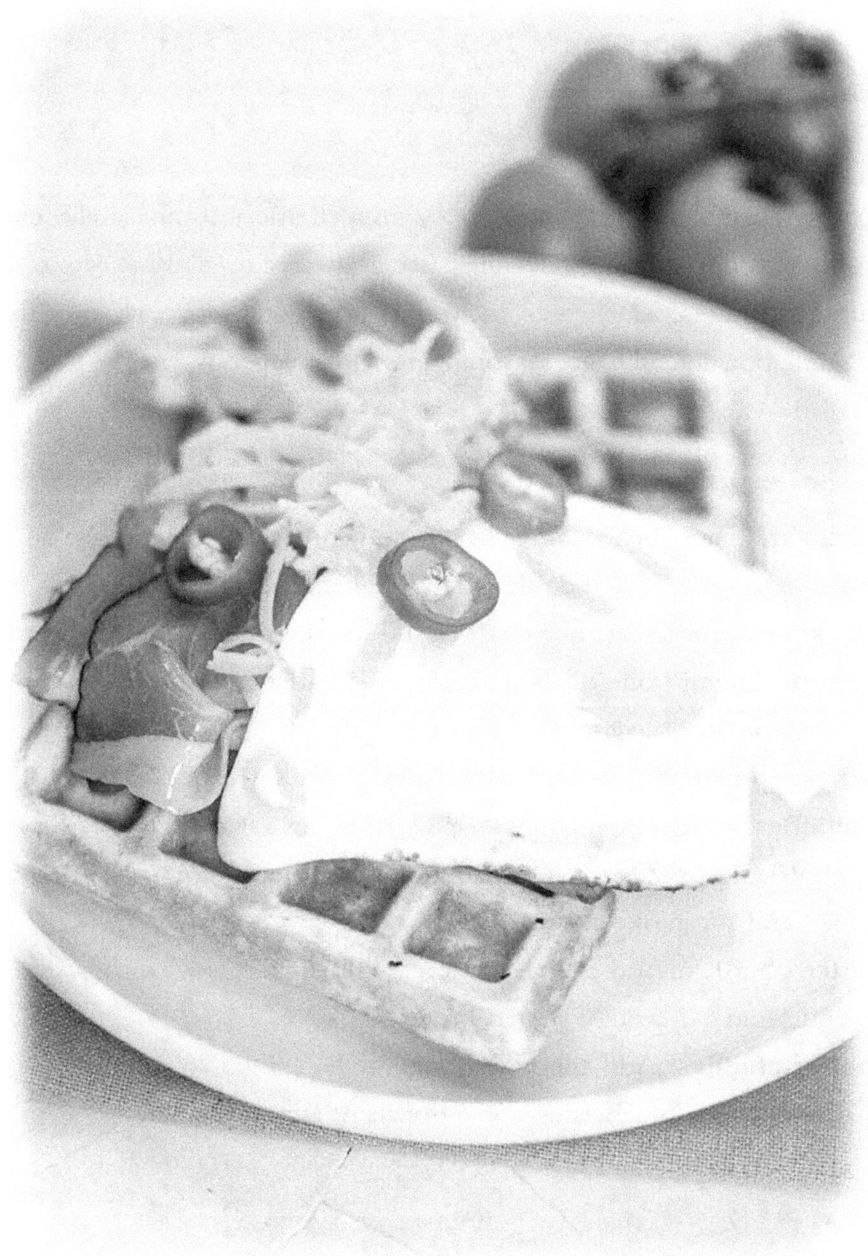

Cheddar, mozzarella, parmesan, cream cheddar, and Colby jack - any cheddar that melts well will work with a chaffle. Distinctive cheddar produces different flavors and somewhat various surfaces. Attempt a couple and locate your top choice.

Following some of the most used:

- **Blue Cheese:** a small crumble of blue cheese contains (1/3 oz.) has 32 calories, 0.2 g of carbs, 2 g of protein, and 2.5 g of fat. Blue cheese is produced from cow, goat, or sheep's milk
- **Feta Cheese:** is made of goat's milk, which can make it easier on the stomach, even for people who are allergic to cow's milk cheese. ¼ cup of crumbled feta cheese gives 1.5 grams of carbs (none of that is fiber, so it's 1.5 grams net). It is a soft, salty, white cheese. It is made from sheep's or goat's milk. Feta gotten from sheep, has a tangy and sharp taste while the one from goat, is milder. It can be used in making chaffles or crumpled over chaffles.
- **Brie Cheese:** is very high in fat and also melty and delicious on almost everything. It contains 0.1 grams of carbs, 6 grams of protein, and 8 grams of fat per 1 ounce. It is a keto-friendly cheese that can be used in making chaffles.
- **Cream Cheese:** this is a keto favorite mainly because the only thing it adds is mostly fat. One tbsp. contains 0.8 g of carbs, less than 1 g of protein, but 5 grams of fat, which shows that it is a great addition to a meal or snack when you need more fat. It can also be served with various keto-friendly vegetables.
- **Paneer:** is a staple cheese, especially in Indian food. About 1-inch cube of Paneer contains 1 gram of carbs, along with 6 grams of protein and 7 grams of fat.
- **Cheese Curds:** are tasty low-carb snacks in their own right but can also be used in making low-carb diets like chaffles. Besides being used in making chaffles or as toppings for chaffles, cheese curds can be used to make a keto-friendly breading out of almond meal and some egg, coated, and fried. It can also be used at the very end of the cooking period with any kind of roasted vegetables, like broccoli or cauliflower (use keto-friendly vegetables).
- **Mozzarella Cheese:** is among the best cheese varieties for a keto diet. 1 serving of Mozzarella cheese contains 0.6 g net carb, 7 g protein, and 6 g fat. It also contains bacteria that act as probiotics, improving gut health, promoting immunity, and fighting inflammation in the body. It is a traditionally southern Italian cheese made from Italian buffalo's milk. Mozzarella cheese has a milky sweetness, which makes it great for various cooking, including chaffles. Mozzarella cheese has a mild enough flavor for sweet chaffles. It is a soft, white cheese with high moisture content.

- **Cheddar Cheese:** it is a relatively hard cheese with a hard texture. It can be sprinkled atop of chaffles or melted into a dip. 1 oz. of cheddar cheese contains 0.1 g carb, 7 g protein, and 9 g of fat. Its taste depends on the variety, ranging from mild to extra sharp. It is a good source of vitamin K, which is important for heart and bone health.
- **Swiss Cheese:** originated from Switzerland; it is a semi-hard cheese made from cow's milk and has a mild, nutty taste. 28 g/1 oz. contains less than 1 g carb, 8 g of protein, and 9 g fat. Its sodium content is more than in most cheeses and offers compounds that may help lower blood pressure.
- **Mascarpone Cheese:** a quality achieved by its especially high percentage of saturated fat. 1 oz of mascarpone cheese contains 0.5 g carb, 13 g fat, and 2 g protein.
- **Ricotta Cheese:** contains 13 g fat, 11 g protein, and 3 g carbohydrate. It is technically made from cow´s milk, sheep, goats, or water buffalo. The use of creamy ricotta cheese keeps the chaffles moist on the inside.
- Other cheese suitable for making chaffles include Tilsit, Roquefort, and Gouda.

TIPS

Caution is required in eating some higher-carb cheeses like:

- Cottage cheese, which contains 5–6 grams of carbs per half a cup.
- Labneh and any other similar yogurt cheeses contain about 4–5 grams per serving, depending on the brand and exact style.

Go for full-fat versions of cheeses where possible, and always watch out for packaged shredded cheeses because some of them have anti-caking agents that add carbs to the total.

EXQUISITE CHAFFLES

Include exquisite fixings like herbs and flavors to your chaffle. For a pizza chaffle, include oregano, garlic powder, and diced pepperoni in the player, with tomato sauce and additional cheddar on top. You could then utilize cream cheddar and add everything bagel flavoring to the player for everything bagel chaffle. Present with more cream cheddar on top, tricks, onions, and smoked salmon.

Check out chaffles and concoct your preferred varieties. They're a fantastic expansion to a ketogenic diet and a great deal of enjoyable to try different things within the kitchen and motivation and progressively great keto food.

What else changes? Sugar yearnings become non-existent after the initial months, Lehner-Gulotta reports. Her patients disclose to her that they feel increasingly fulfilled after dinners, and they're not constantly ravenous.

CHAFFLES VS. WAFFLES

A chaffle is a keto waffle. It's called a chaffle because one of its primary ingredients is shredded cheese, hence the Chaffle instead of Waffle because chaffles are cheese waffles. Pretty cool, right?

Waffles are usually made of flour-based batter, but a chaffle is made of eggs and cheese. It sounds odd, but it actually works!

Chaffles are a great way for those on the keto diet to get their waffle fix. They're also a great way to eat fewer carbs while still eating what you want! Even if it is a modified version. There are also endless chaffle ingredient combinations.

HOW A BASIC CHAFFLE IS MADE

A basic chaffle is made of just two ingredients: ½ cup of shredded cheese, like mozzarella, and 1 large egg. Finely shredded cheese or thicker shreds work; it's completely up to you.

You whisk the egg, stir in the cheese, and place half the mixture in a waffle maker at a time for 2–3 minutes. Then, after removing them from the waffle maker, let them sit for 1–2 minutes. They'll crisp up like a normal waffle would as they set.

You can add almond or coconut flour to give it a more bread-like texture. One teaspoon of either is a good place to start and adjust to your preferences.

HOW TO EAT/SERVE A BASIC CHAFFLE

Even though they are as simple as they can get, there are a lot of ways to eat chaffles:

- **Plain:**
Chaffles are great as a breakfast food on their own. You can serve them up alongside bacon, avocado, eggs, and other standard keto breakfast foods.

- **Keto chaffle sandwich:**

You can make two chaffles and use them to replace the bread for your favorite sandwich. Chaffles are great as the bread for breakfast sandwiches, turkey clubs, or any other keto-friendly sandwiches.

- **Chaffle dessert:**

You can try a sweet chaffle variation and serve it with your favorite keto ice cream or keto maple syrup.

You can also customize your chaffle in all kinds of ways:

- **Different cheeses:**

Mozzarella, Cheddar, Parmesan, Colby Jack, Philadelphia cream cheese—any cheese that melts well will work with a chaffle. Different cheeses produce slightly different textures and different flavors.

- **Sweeteners:**

You can add your favorite keto sweetener, like stevia or sucralose, to the batter before you fry it up. You can also try putting some chocolate chips or low-sugar fruits like strawberries or blueberries.

- **Herbs and spices:**

Put some savory ingredients such as herbs and spices into your chaffle. For a pizza chaffle, sprinkle some oregano, garlic powder, and diced pepperoni into the batter, with tomato sauce and extra cheese on top. Or also, try some cream cheese and add everything bagel seasoning to the batter for everything bagel chaffle. Topped it with more cream cheese, capers, onions, and smoked salmon.

Give chaffles a chance and come up with your own favorite variations. They're an excellent addition to a Ketogenic diet and a lot of fun to experiment with within the kitchen. And for inspiration and more awesome keto food, check out all our low-carb recipes.

Chapter 4.
KETO CHAFFLES PREPARATION

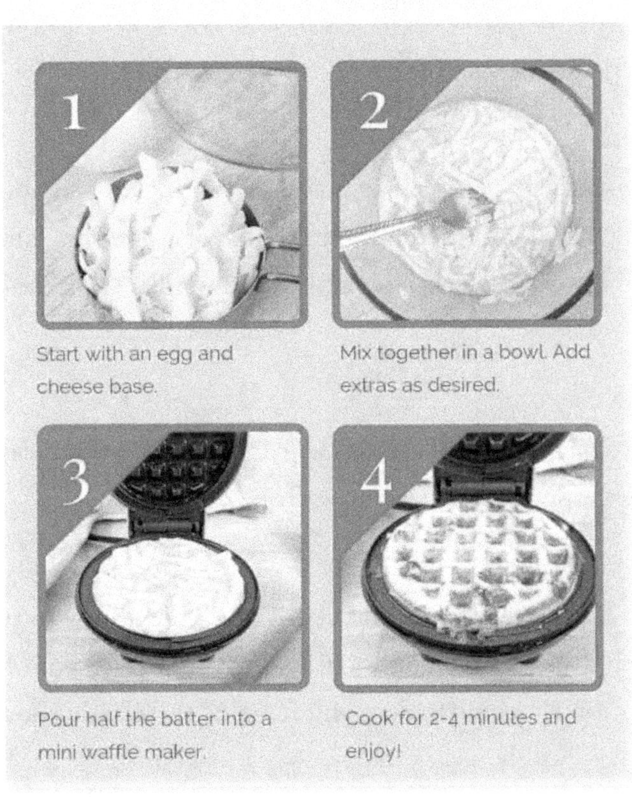

HOW TO MAKE CHAFFLES?

You can prepare chaffles in various flavors and forms using different combinations of ingredients with cheese and eggs, and most of them are extensively covered in the recipe part of the cookbook. Here we shall see how you can make the basic chaffle batter.

- Use finely shredded cheese
- Chaffle batter mixing
- Use a waffle iron to make the chaffle
- Try different toppings

A chaffle maker and a waffle maker are actually the same things. It is a simple appliance that lets you create amazing treats, and there is a wide range of different models and products intended to bring you the fluffiest chaffles and waffles possible.

You might not think of it, but the world of waffle-chaffle makers can be quite vast, with a number of different types to choose from. Because there are that many different types of chaffles and waffles, the devices used to create them also have to be different.

Here are just some of the separate things that are worth considering:

- **Output:**

Output refers to how many waffles at a time the machine can make, and your choice should depend on how many people you have to feed and their appetite. Most standard machines produce just one or two waffles. However, some of them can make up to eight waffles and even beyond in commercial-style waffle makers.

- **Waffle style:**

Waffles come in many different styles, from classic Belgian waffles to traditional American waffles, so you have many specific styles of waffle makers to choose from.

- **Shape:**

Fancy waffle maker's shapes were a bestseller in recent years. The ability to transform your favorite treat into a star or heart was such a hit! These come either as an insert to your waffle maker, or a separate machine. But the most common shape nowadays still remains the classic square or a circle.

- **Thickness:**

You can pick a waffle maker depending on how thick you like your waffles. Most waffles range from thin, of around ½ inch, to thick, of around 1 ½ inch.

- **Grill surface:**

Look for a non-stick grill surface, preferably something coated with Teflon or just made from ceramic. This will help in two ways: your waffles won't stick when you try to get them, and, consequently, the cleanup will be considerably easier.

- **Lights and display:**

Most modern machines have at least a small light indicator that shows when the waffle maker is heated up and ready to cook the batter. More advanced models might also feature another light to show when your waffle is approximately done and even a digital display for further information.

- **Digital timer:**

If you don't use a timer in waffle making, you are more prone to end up under or overcooking your waffle. Both are usually too hard to enjoy, but undercooked waffles additionally stick in the griddle, becoming a mess to dig out! To prevent all of this, some waffle makers have convenient built-in countdown timers.

- **Flip ability:**

Traditionally, flip waffle makers were usually qualified as professionals only, which was making them quite expensive. However, nowadays, there are many new affordable designs with a flip function. They help to achieve an even spread of batter on the grill.

There are many smaller features that might attract some users, such as browning settings and drip trays. However, they are all optional and not necessary.

Thankfully, the range of today's waffle makers is more diverse and accessible than ever before! The choices are all quite enticing. Shop smart and think about what you really want from your waffle maker before pulling the trigger.

MAIN INGREDIENTS TO USE

When you start cooking recipes for a ketogenic diet, one of the most difficult challenges is finding low-carbohydrate ingredients. The bigger problem is when you have to bake bread, cakes, cookies, and similar foods.

Usually, for these purposes, we use wheat flour that gives baked goods the texture we love so much. But, unfortunately, wheat flour, in all its variations, has a very high carbohydrate content that can reach over 75 grams per 100 grams of the product. You can imagine how this is absolutely keto-unfriendly!

- **Almond Flour:**

Almond flour is also gluten-free, which is very appreciated by those who have celiac disease or are intolerant. Of course, gluten is very important because it allows the dough to obtain that adorable soft consistency, and its lack is noticeable during baking.

However, with some simple tricks, you can overcome the problem. For example:

Replace the wheat flour with the same amount of almond flour (so ratio 1:1).

Increase the amount of leavening agent since the specific weight of almond flour is higher than that of classic multipurpose flour.

Use less liquid in recipes to balance the greater volume.

- **Almond Meal:**

It is a variant obtained using unpeeled almonds. Compared to almond flour, it will have a darker color and a coarser texture. It should be used in the same way as almond flour, and the same indications apply as in the paragraph above.

- **Coconut Flour:**

Coconut products are becoming more and more known on the market; it is no surprise that coconut flour is becoming more popular as well. Coconut flour is created from the coconut's inside meat being dried and ground into a fine powder. This specific type of flour has healthy fats, high in protein, and low in carbohydrates. If you have a nut allergy, wheat allergy, or diabetes, coconut flour will be an excellent alternative for your baking needs. You should know before purchasing coconut flour because it is typically sweet from the coconut. It also has a strong scent of coconut and typically has a finer texture compared to other flours. If you do not like coconut, this taste can be hard to mask. However, this flour is excellent for bread, brownies, and cinnamon buns.

- **Nut Flours:**

Nut flours are derived from a variety of nuts (raw or dried) ground to a fine powder. Nut flours bring texture and moisture due to the nuts themselves' oils and bring about a rich taste. Notable nut flour variants, in addition to the already mentioned almond and coconut flour, are hazelnuts, chestnut, pecans, macadamias… but, as I said, I prefer almond flour.

- **Oat Fibers:**

Practically oat fibers consist only of ground husks and are generally not used as the main ingredient for baking. The product obtained by grinding the hull is made up of over 90% insoluble fibers and is practically free of carbohydrates and calories.

Oat fibers also help intestinal regularity and are gluten-free.

- **Xanthan Gum:**

Before we move onto the fun part of baking, you must learn that xanthan gum is going to be your new best friend. You may not recognize this, but many of the gluten-free flour alternatives lack a binding agent.

A binding agent is helpful to hold your food together, much like gluten does when used in baking and cooking. The moment you remove gluten, all mixtures will typically crumble and fall apart. Xanthan gum is made from lactose, sucrose, and glucose that have been fermented from a specific bacterium. When this is added to liquid, it creates a gum and is used with gluten-free baking. As a general guide, you will be using one teaspoon of xanthan gum for one cup of gluten-free flour that you use. For some mixes, this gum is already added, so you will always want to check the ingredient label when you are baking. Keep in mind that xanthan gum can be expensive, but it will last you a long time.

- **All-purpose Keto Flour:**

Cooking is nice, but sometimes you're in a hurry and don't have time to do the calculations to replace classic wheat flour with low-carb alternatives.

So, I came up with this mixture obtained with:

- 1 ½ cup almond flour
- ½ cup coconut flour
- ¼ cup oat fiber
- ¼ cup xanthan gum

Just store it in a cool, dry place and use it instead of regular flour.

If you don't like oat fibers, you can replace them with same amount of xanthan gum.

- **Low Carb Baking Mix:**

If you really don't have time and you don't have any alternative flours with you, the low-carb baking mixes can be just right for you.

Some of the most famous and easiest to buy online (also on Amazon) are:

- Keto and Co Pancake and Waffle Mix
- Julian Bakery Paleo Thin® Pancake & Waffle Mix
- Carbquik

KITCHEN TOOLS TO USE

In order to start preparing your Keto Chaffles or Waffles, you need to learn a few basic dough-making techniques and some simple tools. Some of these tools are probably already in your kitchen.

- **Waffle Maker:**

Obviously, this is an indispensable tool you can't do without. What Kind of Waffle Maker to Use for Chaffles? A mini waffle iron is perfect for making chaffles as it produces the ideal size (4 inches to be exact), cooks them fast, and crisps them up. If you do not have one yet, always pick one with a non-stick coating but chemical-free. The Dash mini waffle maker has recently been gaining popularity in the internet world.

- **Batter Cups:**

Usually supplied together with the waffle maker, the batter cup is a simple gradated plastic container which, when filled to the indicated level, avoids pouring too much dough into the waffle maker, making it overflow.

It will help you not to dirty the kitchen. Each batter cup is specific to its waffle maker model.

- **Batter Dispensers:**

Just like batter cups, batter dispensers are just another way to efficiently pour batter onto the grids of your waffle maker. These serve to cut down on waste by reducing dripping and splattering during pouring, and they also help you have consistent results.

- **Bowls:**

I love using the large metal mixing bowl that I found at a restaurant supply store, but any bowl will do. Make sure you have a variety of sizes so you can measure out different quantities of ingredients. Whenever I shop at thrift stores, I like finding small bowls for a few cents here and there to add to my collection. Having little bowls for ingredients in smaller amounts, like salt, yeast, chopped herbs, and so on, is nice, but it's not absolutely necessary—any vessel will do.

- **Dough Scraper :**

I recommend getting metal and a plastic dough scraper. They cost just a few dollars at kitchen stores, restaurant supply stores, or Amazon, and they are so useful. A metal scraper helps cut and scrape the dough off your work area, and a plastic scraper is flexible enough to help scrape the dough out of the bowl after rinsing.

- **Kitchen Scale:**

Almost all of the ingredients in the recipes are measured in grams, so you will need a kitchen scale that weighs in metrics. Weighing your ingredients is the best way to get the most consistent results in your baking, and once you get used to weighing your ingredients, I promise you won't want to go back. It is so much simpler and makes a huge difference in the final loaf of bread. Kitchen scales are relatively inexpensive these days; small ones can be found for around \$20. They typically have a "mode" button that will easily switch them from ounces to grams.

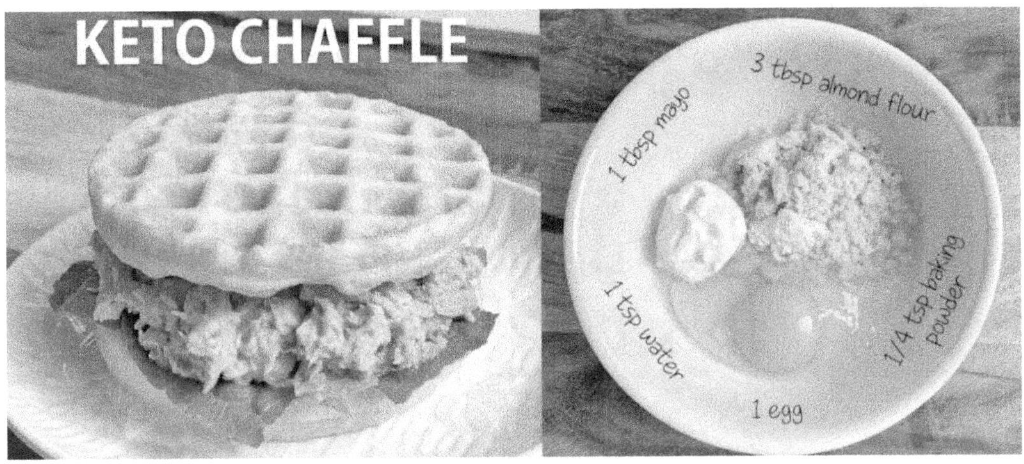

Chapter 5.
FAQS

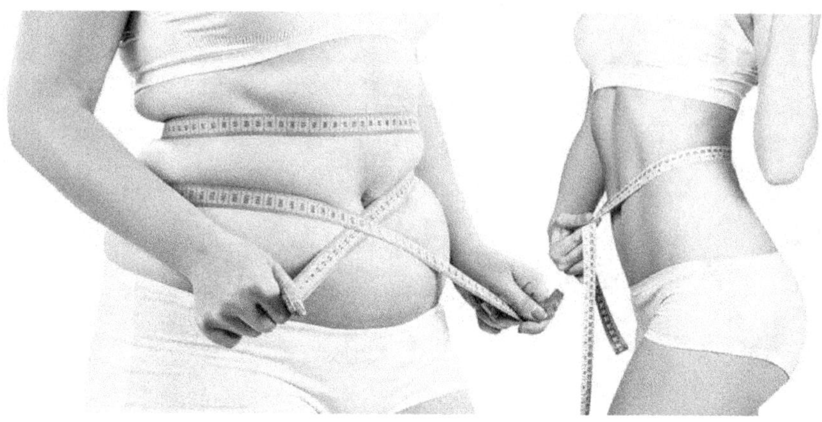

A few questions about chaffles are frequently asked here. Here are responses to some of the most popular ketogenic diet-related questions.

WHAT IS THE BEST CHEESE TO MAKE CHAFFLE?

Oh, another interesting question. Today, we usually use classic, neutral flavors. The choice of cheese actually depends on the flavor. If you're making low-carb bread, you want to chaffle the ancillary actors instead of the reeds.

So, the best cheese for that is mozzarella cheese. I like to use finely ground ones. Because it mixes a little better with the egg, and I generally like to shred my cheese, but the pre-shreds work very well here and add to the useful factors.

Yes, you can use many other slices of cheese, but if you want the cheese to shine, you should. The world is your oyster! Enjoy! And experiment!

Am I Going to Lose my Muscles?

There is a possibility that any diet will lose any muscle. Nevertheless, a high intake of protein and high levels of ketone can help to reduce muscle loss, particularly when lifting weights.

Can I Use a Ketogenic Diet to Build Muscle?

Yes, but a moderate-carb diet may not perform as well. Read in this book and other articles for more information on low-carb diets and exercise efficiency.

Do I Need Carburization or Refeed?

No. No. No. Nonetheless, every now and then, a couple of higher-calorie days may be helpful.

What if I'm tired or weak at all times?

You may not be in full ketosis to make efficient use of fats and ketones. To counter this, raising the consumption of carb and recalling the above points may also help a supplement such as MCT oil or ketones.

My Pee Has a Fruity Scent. Why is it?

Don't worry. This is simply due to the excretion during ketosis of by-products.

The Scent of the Breath. What am I Going to Do?

It's a common side effect. Try to drink flavored water naturally or to chew sugar-free gum.

I Read that Ketosis was Very Risky. Is it True?

Ketosis is often associated with ketoacidosis by men. The former is normal, whereas, in uncontrolled diabetes, the latter happens only.

Ketoacidosis is risky, but it is perfectly normal and healthy to have ketogenic diet ketosis.

I'm Having Problems with Digestion and Diarrhea. What am I Going to Do?

Generally, after 3–4 weeks, this common side effect disappears. If it continues, try to eat more vegetables of high fiber. Constipation can also be helped by magnesium supplements.

Do You Just Taste Chaffles Like Eggs and Cheese?

While plain chaffles can taste like eggs and cheese, with just about any flavor, you can customize chaffles. Using a mild cheese such as mozzarella can eliminate much of the taste of cheese and eggs, leaving you with a blank canvas to fill up as you see fit.

Why Does Chaffle Get Stuck On the Grill?

This happens when the griddle does not cook the chaffle long enough. The dough is not completely cooked before lifting or trying to remove it, and the dough remains stuck to the outside when the griddle is opened. I think it's best to cook most chaffle recipes for at least 3-4 minutes.

It is recommended to cook a chaffle recipe for at least 3–4 minutes. For basic cream cheese, eggs, and cheese dough, you can get away in at least 3 minutes. In some cases, if chicken or tuna are included in the recipe, they need to be cooked longer. Based on the recipe, the cooking time for protein-based chaffles is 4–7 minutes.

Without a Waffle Maker, Would You Make Chaffles?

Without a waffle iron, it's hard to get the crispiness of the chaffles. That said, in a pan that holds a lot of heat, like a cast iron, you should try to mix up the chaffle batter and cook it like a pancake. You probably won't end up with a perfect, standardized end result, but it's still going to be pretty good.

Can You Use Chaffles to Freeze?

You will freeze chaffles up to a month. Defrosting them, though, adds a lot of moisture, making it hard to get them crisp again. Because they're so fast and easy to produce (the overall cooking time is less than 10 minutes), you're probably better off making up a fresh batch whenever you're feeling like a chaffle.

If you are planning to make and reheat the chaffles in advance, you might want to invest in an air fryer. Once they have been in a fridge or freezer, it can be difficult to get chaffles crispy again. In just a few minutes, an air fryer will dehydrate them and crisp them up nicely.

You can cook the chaffles 1–2 minutes per side in a dry pan, or you can position them in a 300-degree Fahrenheit oven for 3-4 minutes or until they are cooked clean. They probably won't get crispy, though, because they are going to retain too much humidity. If you don't have an air fryer, making smaller batches of chaffles and enjoying them fresh is your best bet. This means they're going to be tastier.

Chapter 6.

BASIC CHAFFLE RECIPES

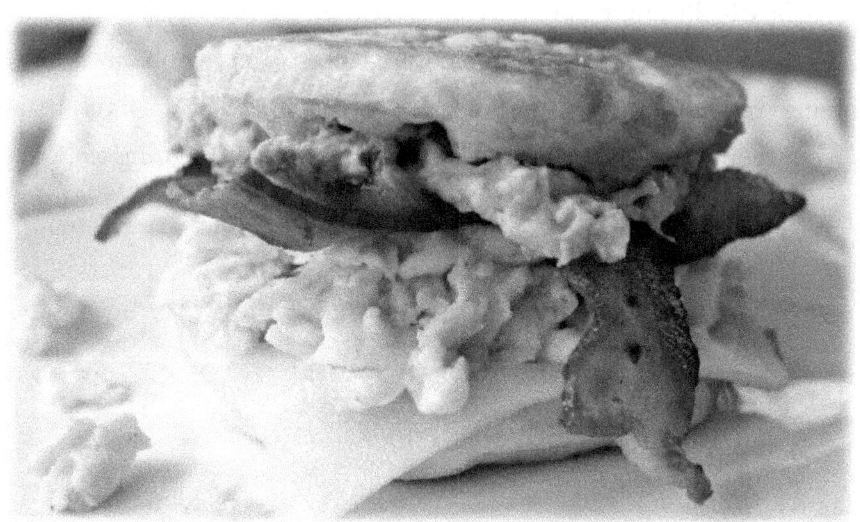

1. BASIC SAVORY CHAFFLES

Preparation Time: 5 minutes

Cooking Time: 7 minutes

Servings: 2

Ingredients:

- 1 large egg
- ½ cup grated Cheddar cheese
- ¼ cup almond flour
- ¼ tsp. gluten-free baking powder

Directions:

1. Preheat the mini waffle maker.
2. Using a blender, mix all the ingredients and blend until smooth.
3. Scoop ½ of the batter into the preheated waffle maker. Close the waffle maker and cook for 3 to 4 minutes.

4. When done, open the lid and let it cool down for 15 to 30 seconds. The chaffle will firm up as it cools. Use a spatula to transfer the chaffle onto a cooling rack. Repeat to make the second chaffle.

5. When still warm, the chaffles will be soft. They will crisp up when completely cooled.

6. Serve immediately or keep in a sealed container at room temperature for up to 3 days, or in the refrigerator for up to 1 week.

Nutrition:

- **Calories**: 225
- **Fat**: 18.5 g
- **Protein**: 12.4 g
- **Carbohydrates**: 9 g

Preparation Time: 5 minutes

Cooking Time: 12 minutes

Servings: 3

Ingredients:

- 1 large egg
- ½ cup grated Mozzarella cheese
- ¼ cup almond flour
- 1/8 tsp. gluten-free baking powder
- 3 tbsp. Swerve

Directions:

1. Preheat the mini waffle maker.
2. Using a blender, mix all the ingredients and blend until smooth.
3. Scoop 1/3 of the batter into the preheated waffle maker. Add them to the center as it spreads. Close the waffle maker and cook for 2 to 4 minutes, checking the waffles after 2 minutes. Keep an eye on the batter in case it overflows.
4. When done, open the lid and let it cool down for 15 to 30 seconds. The chaffle will firm up as it cools. Use a spatula to gently transfer the chaffle onto a cooling rack. Repeat with the remaining batter.
5. When still warm, the chaffles will be soft. They will crisp up when completely cooled.
6. Serve immediately or keep in a sealed container at room temperature for up to 3 days, or in the refrigerator for up to 1 week.

Nutrition:

- **Calories:** 132
- **Fat:** 9.8 g
- **Protein:** 8.4 g
- **Carbohydrates:** 15 g

3. Fluffy White Chaffles

Preparation Time: 10 minutes

Cooking Time: 7 minutes

Servings: 4

Ingredients:

- 1 large egg
- 1 large egg white
- 2 tbsp. cream cheese
- ½ cup grated Mozzarella cheese
- 2 tbsp. coconut flour
- ¼ cup almond flour
- ¼ tsp. vanilla extract
- ½ tsp. baking powder
- ¼ cup Swerve

Directions:

1. Preheat the mini waffle maker.
2. Place the egg, egg white, cream cheese, and Mozzarella into a blender. Process until smooth. Add the remaining ingredients and process again.
3. Spoon one-quarter of the batter into the waffle maker. Cook for 2 to 4 minutes or until golden brown. Transfer the chaffle onto a cooling rack to cool. Repeat with the remaining batter.
4. Serve immediately.

Nutrition:

- **Calories:** 136
- **Fat:** 10.0 g
- **Protein:** 8.4 g
- **Carbohydrates:** 26 g

Preparation Time: 11 minutes

Cooking Time: 6 minutes

Servings: 4

Ingredients:

- 1 large egg
- 1 large egg white
- 2 tbsp. cream cheese
- ½ cup grated Mozzarella cheese
- 2 tbsp. coconut flour
- 2 tbsp. cacao powder
- ½ tsp. baking powder
- ¼ cup Swerve

Directions:

1. Preheat the mini waffle maker.
2. Place the egg, egg white, cream cheese, and Mozzarella into a blender. Process until smooth. Add the remaining ingredients and process again.
3. Spoon one-quarter of the batter into the waffle maker. Cook for 2 to 4 minutes or until golden brown. Transfer the chaffle onto a cooling rack to cool. Repeat with the remaining batter.
4. Serve immediately.

Nutrition:

- **Calories**: 106
- **Fat**: 7.1 g
- **Protein**: 7.6 g
- **Carbohydrates**: 6 g

5. BLUEBERRY KETO CHAFFLE

Preparation Time: 5 minutes

Cooking Time: 17 minutes

Servings: 5

Ingredients:

- 2 eggs
- 1 cup Mozzarella cheese
- 2 tbsp. almond flour
- 2 tsp. Swerve, plus additional for serving
- 1 tsp. baking powder
- 1 tsp. cinnamon
- 3 tbsp. blueberries
- Nonstick cooking spray

Directions:

1. Preheat the mini waffle maker.
2. Stir together the eggs, Mozzarella cheese, almond flour, swerve, baking powder, cinnamon, and blueberries in a mixing bowl. Brush the waffle maker with nonstick cooking spray.
3. Pour in a little bit less than ¼ a cup of blueberry waffle batter at a time.
4. Seal the lid and cook the chaffle for 3 to 5 minutes. Check it at the 3-minute mark to see if it is crispy and brown. If not or it sticks to the top of the waffle maker, close the lid and cook for an additional 1 to 2 minutes.
5. Serve sprinkled with additional Swerve.

Nutrition:

- **Calories:** 120
- **Fat:** 8.3 g
- **Protein:** 8.4 g
- **Carbohydrates:** 7 g

Preparation Time: 5 minutes

Cooking Time: 21 minutes

Servings: 5

Ingredients:

- 2 eggs, beaten
- 1 cup taco blend cheese
- 1 tbsp. almond flour
- ¼ tsp. taco seasoning

Directions:

1. Preheat the mini waffle maker.
2. Mix all the ingredients, then stir until well incorporated.
3. Pour 1½ tbsp. of batter into the waffle maker at a time. Cook for 4 minutes.
4. Remove the taco chaffle shell from the waffle maker and drape it over the side of a bowl. Continue making chaffle taco shells until you are out of batter.
5. Fill the taco shells with your favorite toppings and serve.

Nutrition:

- **Calories:** 115
- **Fat:** 9.2 g
- **Protein:** 8.3 g
- **Carbohydrates:** 4 g

Preparation Time: 5 minutes

Cooking Time: 11 minutes

Servings: 2

Ingredients:

- 1 egg
- ¾ cup shredded Mozzarella cheese, divided
- 1 tbsp. almond flour
- ½ tsp. basil
- ½ tsp. garlic powder, divided
- 1 tbsp. butter

Directions:

1. Preheat the mini waffle maker.
2. Stir together the egg, ½ cup of cheese, almond flour, basil, and ¼ tsp. of garlic powder in a small bowl.
3. Fill in half of the batter into your mini waffle maker and cook for 4 minutes. If they are still a bit uncooked, leave it cooking for an additional 2 minutes. Repeat with the remaining batter.
4. In a small bowl, add the butter and remaining ¼ tsp. of garlic powder and melt in the microwave, about 25 seconds.
5. Arrange the chaffles on a baking sheet and spread the butter mixture on top. Scatter each chaffle with 1/8 cup of cheese.
6. Put the chaffles in the oven or a toaster oven at 400°F (205°C) and cook until the cheese melts.
7. Cool for 5 minutes before serving.

Nutrition:

- **Calories:** 233
- **Fat:** 19.3 g
- **Protein:** 13.3 g
- **Carbohydrates:** 16 g

Preparation Time: 5 minutes

Cooking Time: 8 minutes

Servings: 2

Ingredients:

- 1 egg, beaten
- ½ cup shredded Mozzarella cheese
- 3 tbsp. Swerve
- 2 tbsp. peanut butter

Directions:

1. Preheat the mini waffle maker.
2. Incorporate all the ingredients, then stir until well incorporated.
3. Fill in half of the batter into the waffle maker and cook for 4 minutes.
4. Transfer to a plate to cool. The chaffle will be a little flimsy when you remove it, but it will stiffen up as it cools. Repeat with the remaining batter.
5. Serve warm.

Nutrition:

- **Calories**: 213
- **Fat**: 16.3 g
- **Protein**: 13 g
- **Carbohydrates**: 6 g

Preparation Time: 2 minutes

Cooking Time: 7 minutes

Servings: 2

Ingredients:

- 1 egg
- 2 tbsp. creamy peanut butter
- ¼ cup shredded Mozzarella cheese
- 1 tbsp. Swerve, plus additional for serving
- 1 tbsp. almond flour
- 1 tsp. vanilla extract
- 1 tbsp. low-carb chocolate chips

Directions:

1. Preheat the mini waffle maker.
2. Whisk the egg and the peanut butter until combined.
3. Whisk in the Mozzarella cheese, Swerve, almond flour, vanilla, and chocolate chips and mix well.
4. Fill in half of the mixture into the waffle maker at a time and cook for 4 minutes.
5. Serve with a sprinkle of Swerve.

Nutrition:

- **Calories**: 195
- **Fat**: 15.1 g
- **Protein**: 11.4 g
- **Carbohydrates**: 8 g

Preparation Time: 2 minutes

Cooking Time: 8 minutes

Servings: 2

Ingredients:

- 1 egg
- ½ cup Cheddar cheese
- ¼ cup chopped fresh broccoli
- 1 tbsp. almond flour
- ¼ tsp. garlic powder

Directions:

1. Mix all the ingredients until completely mixed.
2. Fill in half of the batter into the waffle maker at a time. Cook for 4 minutes.
3. Let cool for 1 to 2 minutes before serving.

Nutrition:

- **Calories**: 174
- **Fat**: 13.2 g
- **Protein**: 11.4 g
- **Carbohydrates**: 14 g

Preparation Time: 5 minutes

Cooking Time: 8 minutes

Servings: 2

Ingredients:

- 1 egg, beaten
- 2 tbsp. cocoa
- 2 tbsp. shredded Mozzarella cheese
- 2 tbsp. Swerve
- 1 tsp. heavy whipping cream
- 1 tsp. coconut flour
- ¼ tsp. vanilla extract
- ¼ tsp. baking powder
- Pinch salt
- Cooking spray

Directions:

1. Preheat the mini waffle maker. Lightly spray it with cooking spray.
2. Mix remaining ingredients, then stir to incorporate.
3. Fill in half of the batter into the waffle maker. Close the lid and cook for 4 minutes. Transfer to a plate and repeat with the remaining batter.
4. Serve hot.

Nutrition:

- **Calories:** 113
- **Fat:** 7.3 g
- **Protein:** 7.2 g
- **Carbohydrates:** 6 g

Preparation Time: 5 minutes

Cooking Time: 8 minutes

Servings: 2

Ingredients:

- 1 egg
- ½ cup Mozzarella cheese
- 1 tbsp. cream cheese, softened
- 1 tbsp. Swerve, plus more for serving
- ¼ tsp. sugar-free banana extract
- ¼ tsp. vanilla extract
- Chopped pecans, for serving

Directions:

1. Preheat the mini waffle maker.
2. Whip the egg in a small bowl. Stir in remaining ingredients and stir until well incorporated.
3. Pour half the batter into the waffle maker and cook for a minimum of 4 minutes until golden brown. Transfer to a plate and repeat with the remaining batter.
4. Serve topped with the Swerve and pecans.

Nutrition:

- **Calories:** 116
- **Fat:** 7.9 g
- **Protein:** 8.9 g
- **Carbohydrates:** 5 g

Preparation Time: 5 minutes

Cooking Time: 4 minutes

Servings: 4

Ingredients:

Chaffle Cake:

- 2 ounces (57 g) cream cheese, softened
- 2 eggs
- 2 tbsp. coconut flour
- 2 tsp. butter, melted
- 1 tsp. baking powder
- 1 tsp. Swerve, or more to taste
- ½ tsp. lemon extract
- 20 drops cake batter extract

Chaffle Frosting:

- ½ cup heavy whipping cream
- 1 tbsp. Swerve
- ¼ tsp. lemon extract

Directions:

1. Preheat the mini waffle maker.
2. Place all the ingredients for the chaffle cake in a blender and blend until the mixture is nice and smooth.
3. Use an ice cream scoop (about 3 tbsp.) and fill the waffle maker with one full scoop of batter. Cook each chaffle for 3 to 4 minutes until golden brown.
4. Meanwhile, make the frosting by whisking together all the frosting ingredients in a medium bowl until the frosting is thick with peaks.
5. Let the chaffles cool completely before frosting the cake. Serve immediately.

Nutrition:

- **Calories**: 224
- **Fat**: 20.5 g
- **Protein**: 5.9 g
- **Carbohydrates**: 12 g

Preparation Time: 5 minutes

Cooking Time: 4 minutes

Servings: 2

Ingredients:

Chaffle:

- 1 egg
- ¼ cup almond flour
- 2 tsp. cream cheese, room temperature
- 1 tsp. Swerve
- ½ tsp. baking powder
- ½ tsp. lime extract or 1 tsp. freshly squeezed lime juice
- ½ tsp. lime zest
- Pinch salt

Frosting:

- 4 ounces (113 g) cream cheese, softened
- 4 tbsp. butter
- 2 tsp. Swerve
- 1 tsp. lime extract
- ½ tsp. lime zest

Directions:

1. Preheat the mini waffle maker.
2. Place all the chaffle ingredients in a blender and blend on high until smooth and creamy.
3. Using an ice cream scoop and pour in the waffle maker with one full scoop of batter. Cook each chaffle for about 3 to 4 minutes until golden brown.
4. Meanwhile, make the frosting by whisking together all the frosting ingredients in a small bowl until smooth.
5. Let the chaffles cool completely before frosting them. Serve immediately.

Nutrition:

- **Calories:** 95
- **Fat:** 5.9 g
- **Protein:** 5.7 g
- **Carbohydrates:** 8 g

15. JICAMA HASH BROWN CHAFFLES

Preparation Time: 5 minutes

Cooking Time: 12 minutes

Servings: 4

Ingredients:

- 1 large jicama root, peeled and shredded
- Salt and pepper, to taste
- 2 eggs, whisked
- 1 cup shredded Cheddar cheese
- 2 garlic cloves, crushed
- ½ medium onion, minced

Directions:

1. Sprinkle the shredded jicama in a large colander and season with salt. Allow standing for 5 to 10 minutes. Using your hands, squeeze out as much liquid as possible.
2. Microwave for 5 to 8 minutes. Allow cooling to room temperature.
3. Transfer the jicama to a large bowl, along with the remaining ingredients. Stir to combine well.
4. Sprinkle a little cheese onto the waffle maker before adding the jicama mixture.
5. Pour 3 tbsp. of the mixture into the waffle maker and cook for a minimum of 3 to 4 minutes.
6. Top with a sprinkle of cheese and serve.

Nutrition:

- **Calories:** 168
- **Fat:** 11.9 g
- **Protein:** 10.2 g
- **Carbohydrates:** 8 g

16. CREAM CHEESE PUMPKIN CHAFFLE

Preparation Time: 5 minutes

Cooking Time: 10 minutes

Servings: 3

Ingredients:

- 1 egg
- ½ cup shredded Mozzarella cheese
- 1 tbsp. sugar-free pumpkin purée
- ½ tsp. pumpkin pie spice

Cream Cheese Frosting:

- 2 tbsp. cream cheese, softened
- 2 tbsp. Swerve
- ½ tsp. vanilla extract

Directions:

1. Preheat the mini waffle maker.
2. Whip the egg in a small bowl. Add the cheese, pumpkin pie spice, and pumpkin and stir to mix well.
3. Fill in half of the mixture into the waffle maker, then cook for a minimum of 3 to 4 minutes until golden brown.
4. Meanwhile, whisk together all the cream cheese frosting ingredients until smooth.
5. Pour in cream cheese frosting to the hot chaffle and serve immediately.

Nutrition:

- **Calories:** 86
- **Fat:** 4.7 g
- **Protein:** 6.3 g
- **Carbohydrates:** 2.6 g

17. VANILLA CHAFFLE

Preparation Time: 5 minutes

Cooking Time: 4 minutes

Servings: 4

Ingredients:

- 2 large eggs
- 2 tbsp. butter, melted
- 2 ounces (57 g) cream cheese, softened
- ¼ cup Swerve
- 1 tsp. vanilla extract
- Pinch pink salt
- ¼ cup almond flour
- 2 tbsp. coconut flour
- 1 tsp. baking powder

Directions:

1. Preheat the mini waffle maker.
2. Whisk eggs into the melted butter in a bowl until creamy.
3. Add the cream cheese, Swerve, vanilla, salt, and stir until just incorporated.
4. Add the almond flour, coconut flour, and baking powder and blend until well combined.
5. Spoon 2 tbsp. of batter into the waffle maker at a time and cook for 4 minutes until golden brown.
6. Serve hot.

Nutrition:

- **Calories:** 157
- **Fat:** 9.2 g
- **Protein:** 6.0 g
- **Carbohydrates:** 4 g

18. PEPPERMINT MOCHA CHAFFLES

Preparation Time: 5 minutes

Cooking Time: 4 minutes

Servings: 6

Ingredients:

Chaffles:

- 1 egg
- 1-ounce (28 g) cream cheese, at room temperature
- 2 tbsp. Swerve
- 1 tbsp. unsweetened cocoa powder
- 1 tbsp. melted butter or coconut oil
- 1 tbsp. almond flour
- 1 tsp. instant coffee granules
- 2 tsp. coconut flour
- ¼ tsp. baking powder
- ¼ tsp. vanilla extract
- Pinch salt

Frosting:

- 2 tbsp. butter, at room temperature
- 2 to 3 tbsp. Swerve
- ¼ tsp. vanilla extract
- 1/8 tsp. peppermint extract

Directions:

1. Preheat the mini waffle maker.
2. Beat all the chaffle ingredients together in a small bowl until smooth.
3. Ladle a heaping 2 tbsp. of batter into waffle maker and cook for about 4 minutes until done. Repeat with the remaining batter.
4. Meanwhile, make the frosting: In a small bowl with a hand mixer, beat the butter and Swerve until creamy.

5. Transfer heavy cream and vanilla extract and beat at high speed for about 4 minutes, or until light and fluffy.
6. Spread the frosting on each chaffle and serve warm.

Nutrition:

- **Calories**: 98
- **Fat**: 9.0 g
- **Protein**: 2.1 g
- **Carbohydrates**: 3 g

Preparation Time: 5 minutes

Cooking Time: 5 minutes

Servings: 4

Ingredients:

Chaffles:

- 1 cup shredded zucchini
- 1-ounce (28 g) cream cheese, softened
- 1 egg
- 1 tbsp. plus 1 tsp. erythritol blend
- 2 tsp. melted butter
- 2 tsp. coconut flour
- ½ tsp. baking powder
- ½ tsp. cinnamon
- Dash ground nutmeg
- 3 tbsp. chopped walnuts or pecans

Frosting:

- 2 tbsp. butter, at room temperature
- 2 oz. (57 g) cream cheese, at room temp
- ¼ tsp. cinnamon
- 1 tbsp. Swerve

Directions:

1. Put the shredded zucchini in a colander over a plate to drain for 15 minutes. With your hands, squeeze out as much liquid as possible.
2. Preheat the mini waffle maker.
3. Stir together all chaffle ingredients until mix.
4. Ladle a heaping 2 tbsp. of batter into the waffle maker. Close the lid and cook 3 to 5 minutes until done. Repeat with the remaining batter.
5. Beat all ingredients for the frosting in a small bowl until smooth. Spread the frosting over each chaffle and serve immediately.

Nutrition:

- **Calories**: 190
- **Fat**: 18.4 g
- **Protein**: 3.5 g
- **Carbohydrates**: 8 g

Preparation Time: 5 minutes

Cooking Time: 2 minutes

Servings: 3

Ingredients:

- 1 egg, beaten
- 1 tbsp. cream cheese, softened
- 1 tbsp. almond flour
- 1 tsp. heavy cream
- ½ tbsp. Swerve, plus more for serving
- ¼ tsp. vanilla extract
- Pinch cinnamon

Directions:

1. Preheat the mini griddle.
2. Pulse all ingredients in a small blender until smooth. Let the batter rest for 5 minutes.
3. Pour 1½ tbsp. of batter into the preheated griddle at a time and cook for 30 seconds. Flip with tongs and cook for a few seconds more.
4. Serve with a sprinkle of Swerve.

Nutrition:

- **Calories:** 63
- **Fat:** 4.1 g
- **Protein:** 2.9 g
- **Carbohydrates:** 6.6 g

Preparation Time: 8 minutes

Cooking Time: 7 minutes

Servings: 2

Ingredients:

- Cheddar cheese: 1/3 cup
- Egg: 1
- Spinach: 1/3 cup finely chopped
- Lemon juice: 2 tbsp.
- Almond flour: 2 tbsp.
- Baking powder: ¼ tsp.
- Ground almonds: 2 tbsp.
- Mozzarella cheese: 1/3 cup

Directions:

1. Mix cheddar cheese, egg, lemon juice, spinach, almond flour, almond ground, and baking powder together in a bowl.
2. Preheat your waffle iron and grease it.
3. In your mini waffle iron, shred half of the mozzarella cheese
4. Add the mixture to your mini waffle iron.
5. Again, shred the remaining mozzarella cheese on the mixture.
6. Cook till the desired crisp is achieved.
7. Make as many chaffles as your mixture and waffle maker allow.

Nutrition:

- **Calories:** 342
- **Fat:** 24 g
- **Protein:** 19.7 g
- **Carbohydrates:** 26 g

22. Okra Fritter Chaffle

Preparation Time: 15 minutes

Cooking Time: 7 minutes

Servings: 2

Ingredients:

- 1 egg
- ¼ cup Mozzarella cheese
- ½ tbsp. onion powder
- 2 tbsp. heavy cream
- 1 tbsp. mayo
- 2 cloves garlic (finely chopped)
- ¼ cup almond flour
- 1 cup okra
- ¼ tsp. salt, or to your taste
- ¼ tsp. black pepper or to your taste

Directions:

1. Combine egg, mayo, and heavy cream and whisk.
2. When mixed, add almond flour, and make a uniform batter.
3. Leave it for 5–10 minutes.
4. Now add okra and the rest of the ingredients and mix well.
5. Preheat a mini waffle maker if needed and grease it.
6. Pour the mixture into the lower plate of the waffle maker and spread it evenly to cover the plate properly.
7. Cook for at least 4 minutes to get the desired crunch.
8. Remove the chaffle from the heat.
9. Make as many chaffles as your mixture and waffle maker allow.
10. Serve hot and enjoy!

Nutrition:

- **Calories:** 339
- **Fat:** 28 g
- **Protein:** 19 g
- **Carbohydrates:** 14 g

Preparation Time: 5 minutes

Cooking Time: 10 minutes

Servings: 2

Ingredients:

- 2 eggs
- 1 cup mozzarella, shredded
- 2 tbsp. cream cheese
- 1 tbsp. butter
- ½ cup onion
- ½ cup tomato
- 1 tbsp. garlic powder
- ¼ tsp. pepper
- ½ tsp. basil
- ½ cup spinach, chopped
- 1 cup carrot, sliced
- ¼ tsp. salt

Directions:

1. Take a pan, heat butter, and add onion and sauté for a minute.
2. Add tomatoes, spinach, and carrot and cook for 10 minutes.
3. Preheat your mini waffle iron if needed.
4. Mix all the above-mentioned ingredients in a bowl with carrots and blend using a hand blender.
5. Grease your waffle iron lightly
6. Cook your mixture in the mini waffle iron for at least 4 minutes.
7. Serve hot with your favorite sauce.
8. Make as many chaffles as your mixture and waffle maker allow.

Nutrition:

- **Calories**: 339
- **Fat**: 24 g
- **Protein**: 17 g
- **Carbohydrates**: 9 g

Preparation Time: 5 minutes

Cooking Time: 7 minutes

Servings: 2

Ingredients:

- 1 egg
- ½ cup cheddar cheese, (shredded)
- 1 tsp. thyme
- a pinch allspice
- Salt and pepper to your taste
- ½ cup chopped coriander

Directions:

1. Mix all the ingredients well together.
2. Pour a layer on a preheated waffle iron.
3. Cook the chaffle for around 5 minutes.
4. Make as many chaffles as your mixture and waffle maker allow.

Nutrition:

- **Calories:** 329
- **Fat:** 25 g
- **Protein:** 16 g
- **Carbohydrates:** 5 g

25. Pickled Spinach Chaffles

Preparation Time: 15 minutes

Cooking Time: 7 minutes

Servings: 2

Ingredients:

- 1 egg
- ½ cup spinach chopped, boiled, and drained
- ½ cup Cheddar cheese (shredded)
- ½ cup Pork panko
- 6–8 thin pickle slices

Directions:

1. Mix egg, spinach, cheese, and pork panko.
2. Fill in a thin layer on a preheated waffle iron.
3. Remove any excess juice from pickles.
4. Add pickle slices and pour more mixture again over the top.
5. Cook the chaffle for around 5 minutes.
6. Make as many chaffles as your mixture and waffle maker allow.

Nutrition:

- **Calories:** 394
- **Fat:** 28 g
- **Protein:** 11 g
- **Carbohydrates:** 8 g

Preparation Time: 5 minutes

Cooking Time: 7 minutes

Servings: 2

Ingredients:

- 1 egg
- ½ cup Mozzarella cheese (shredded)
- ½ cup finely grated zucchini
- ½ cup chopped onion
- ½ tsp. garlic powder
- ¼ tsp. pepper
- ¼ tsp. salt

Directions:

1. Preheat a mini waffle maker if needed and grease it.
2. Mix all the ingredients of the chaffle and mix well.
3. Pour the mixture into the waffle maker.
4. Cook for at least 4 minutes to get the desired crunch and make as many chaffles as your batter allows.

Nutrition:

- **Calories:** 341
- **Fat:** 25 g
- **Protein:** 16 g
- **Carbohydrates:** 11 g

Preparation Time: 15 minutes

Cooking Time: 7 minutes

Servings: 4

Ingredients:

- 2 eggs
- 1 cup Cheddar cheese (shredded)
- ¼ cup chopped mint:
- ½ cup onion, chopped
- ½ cup cucumber, chopped
- ½ cup tomato, chopped
- ½ cup lettuce, chopped
- ½ cup cabbage chopped
- ½ tsp. salt
- ¼ tsp. black pepper
- ½ cup fresh coriander, chopped

Directions:

1. Preheat a mini waffle maker if needed and grease it.
2. Whisk eggs and sprinkle mint and shredded cheddar cheese to them.
3. Mix them all well, then fill the mixture to the lower plate of the waffle maker.
4. Cook for at least 4 minutes to get the desired crunch.
5. Remove from the heat and divide into four pieces when cool down.
6. Mix all the vegetable and seasoning and add chaffles too and serve.

Nutrition:

- **Calories**: 331
- **Fat**: 27 g
- **Protein**: 14 g
- **Carbohydrates**: 8 g

Preparation Time: 25 minutes

Cooking Time: 7 minutes

Servings: 4

Ingredients:

- 2 eggs
- ½ cup Mozzarella cheese (shredded)
- 2 tbsp. cream cheese
- 1 cup broccoli
- ½ cup pumpkin puree
- 1 tbsp. butter
- ½ cup onion
- ½ cup tomato
- 1 tbsp. garlic powder
- ¼ tsp. pepper
- ½ tsp. basil
- ¼ tsp. salt

Directions:

1. Take a pan, heat butter, add onion and sauté for a minute.
2. Add tomatoes and broccoli and cook till tender.
3. Preheat your mini waffle iron if needed.
4. Mix all the ingredients mentioned above in a bowl with broccoli and blend using a hand blender.
5. Grease your waffle iron lightly.
6. Cook your mixture in the mini waffle iron for at least 4 minutes.
7. Serve hot with your favorite sauce.
8. Make as many chaffles as your mixture and waffle maker allow.

Nutrition:

- **Calories:** 382
- **Fat:** 21 g
- **Protein:** 12 g
- **Carbohydrates:** 7 g

Preparation Time: 13 minutes

Cooking Time: 7 minutes

Servings: 2

Ingredients:

- 2 eggs
- ½ cup mashed boiled broccoli:
- ½ cup Cheddar cheese (shredded)
- ½ cup pork panko
- 6–8 thin pickle slices

Directions:

1. Mix egg, broccoli, cheese, and pork panko.
2. Fill in a thin layer on a preheated waffle iron.
3. Remove any excess juice from pickles.
4. Add pickle slices and pour more mixture again over the top.
5. Cook the chaffle for around 5 minutes.
6. Make as many chaffles as your mixture and waffle maker allow.

Nutrition:

- **Calories:** 339
- **Fat:** 29 g
- **Protein:** 14 g
- **Carbohydrates:** 6 g

Preparation Time: 5 minutes

Cooking Time: 7 minutes

Servings: 2

Ingredients:

- 1 egg
- ½ cup Mozzarella cheese (shredded)
- 1 tsp. thyme:
- ½ cup radish, finely grated
- A pinch allspice:
- Salt and pepper: to your taste
- ½ cup chopped coriander:

Directions:

1. Mix all the ingredients well together.
2. Pour a layer on a preheated waffle iron.
3. Cook the chaffle for around 5 minutes.
4. Make as many chaffles as your mixture and waffle maker allow.

Nutrition:

- **Calories**: 382
- **Fat**: 31 g
- **Protein**: 21 g
- **Carbohydrates**: 26 g

31. BOILED BROCCOLI MOZZARELLA CHAFFLES

Preparation Time: 25 minutes

Cooking Time: 7 minutes

Servings: 2

Ingredients:

- 2 eggs
- 1 cup Mozzarella cheese (shredded)
- 2 tbsp. cream cheese
- 1 cup broccoli
- ¼ tsp. salt

Directions:

1. Boil broccoli for 15 minutes in salted water.
2. Preheat your mini waffle iron if needed.
3. Mix all the ingredients mentioned above in a bowl with broccoli and blend using a hand blender.
4. Grease your waffle iron lightly.
5. Cook your mixture in the mini waffle iron for at least 4 minutes.
6. Serve hot with your favorite sauce.
7. Make as many chaffles as your mixture and waffle maker allow.

Nutrition:

- **Calories**: 370
- **Fat**: 24 g
- **Protein**: 17 g
- **Carbohydrates**: 16 g

Preparation Time: 5 minutes

Cooking Time: 7 minutes

Servings: 2

Ingredients:

- 1 zucchini (small)
- 1 egg
- ½ cup mozzarella cheese (shredded)
- 1 tbsp. Parmesan
- Pepper to taste
- 1 tsp. basil
- ½ cup spinach

Directions:

1. Preheat your waffle iron.
2. Grate zucchini finely.
3. Boil spinach for five minutes and strain water.
4. Add all the ingredients to zucchini in a bowl and mix well.
5. Now add the spinach.
6. Grease your waffle iron lightly.
7. Pour the mixture into a full-size waffle maker and spread evenly.
8. Cook till it turns crispy.
9. Make as many chaffles as your mixture and waffle maker allow.
10. Serve crispy and with your favorite keto sauce.

Nutrition:

- **Calories:** 391
- **Fat:** 31 g
- **Protein:** 29 g
- **Carbohydrates:** 24 g

Preparation Time: 15 minutes

Cooking Time: 7 minutes

Servings: 2

Ingredients:

- 2 eggs
- 1 cup Mozzarella cheese (shredded)
- 2 tbsp. cream cheese
- 1 tbsp. butter
- ½ cup onion:
- ½ cup tomato
- 1 tbsp. garlic powder
- ¼ tsp. pepper
- ½ tsp. basil
- ½ cup cabbage, finely shredded
- 1 cup carrot, sliced
- ¼ tsp. salt

Directions:

1. Take a pan, heat butter, add onion, and sauté for a minute.
2. Add tomatoes and carrot and cook for 10 minutes.
3. Preheat your mini waffle iron if needed.
4. Mix all the ingredients mentioned above in a bowl with carrots except for cabbage and blend using a hand blender.
5. Add cabbage to the mixture from the top and mix.
6. Grease your waffle iron lightly.
7. Cook your mixture in the mini waffle iron for at least 4 minutes.
8. Serve hot with your favorite sauce.
9. Make as many chaffles as your mixture and waffle maker allow.

Nutrition:

- **Calories:** 388
- **Fat:** 29 g
- **Protein:** 11 g
- **Carbohydrates:** 10 g

Preparation Time: 5 minutes

Cooking Time: 7 minutes

Servings: 2

Ingredients:

- ½ cup cauliflower
- ½ cup okra
- 2 eggs
- 1 cup Mozzarella cheese (shredded)
- 1 tbsp. butter
- 2 tbsp. almond flour
- ¼ tsp. turmeric
- ¼ tsp. baking powder
- A pinch onion powder
- A pinch garlic powder
- A pinch salt

Directions:

1. In a deep saucepan, boil okra and cauliflower for five minutes or till it tenders, strain, and set aside
2. Incorporate all the remaining ingredients, mixing well together
3. Fill in a thin layer on a preheated waffle iron
4. Take out any excess water from the vegetables and add a layer to the mixture
5. Again, add more mixture over the top
6. Cook the chaffle for around 5 minutes
7. Serve hot with your favorite keto sauce

Nutrition:

- **Calories:** 332
- **Fat:** 28.1 g
- **Protein:** 19.7 g
- **Carbohydrates:** 14 g

35. Oniony Pickled Chaffles

Preparation Time: 25 minutes

Cooking Time: 7 minutes

Servings: 2

Ingredients:

- 1 egg
- ½ cup finely chopped onion:
- ½ cup Cheddar cheese (shredded)
- ½ cup pork panko
- 6-8 thin pickle slices
- 1 tbsp. pickle juice

Directions:

1. Mix egg, onion, cheese, and pork panko.
2. Fill in a thin layer on a preheated waffle iron.
3. Remove any excess juice from pickles.
4. Add pickle slices and pour more mixture again over the top.
5. Cook the chaffle for around 5 minutes.
6. Make as many chaffles as your mixture and waffle maker allow.

Nutrition:

- **Calories:** 366
- **Fat:** 27 g
- **Protein:** 10 g
- **Carbohydrates:** 9 g

Preparation Time: 5 minutes

Cooking Time: 7 minutes

Servings: 2

Ingredients:

- 1 egg
- ½ cup Cheddar cheese (shredded)
- 1 tsp. thyme
- ½ cup chopped spinach
- a pinch allspice
- Salt and pepper: to your taste
- ½ cup chopped coriander

Directions:

1. Mix all the ingredients well together.
2. Pour a layer on a preheated waffle iron.
3. Cook the chaffle for around 5 minutes.
4. Make as many chaffles as your mixture and waffle maker allow.

Nutrition:

- **Calories:** 391
- **Fat:** 26 g
- **Protein:** 19.7 g
- **Carbohydrates:** 16 g

37. VEGGIES AND OLIVES CHAFFLES SALAD

Preparation Time: 12 minutes

Cooking Time: 7 minutes

Servings: 2

Ingredients:

- 2 eggs
- 1 cup Cheddar cheese (shredded)
- ½ cup thickly sliced onion
- ½ cup thickly sliced zucchini
- 1 cup florets removed cauliflower
- ½ tsp. salt
- ¼ tsp. black pepper
- 1 tsp. butter
- ½ cup olives, sliced
- ½ cup chopped fresh coriander

Directions:

1. Preheat the oven.
2. Add all the vegetables to the baking tray and sprinkle salt and pepper.
3. Brush with oil and roast for 15 min.
4. Preheat a mini waffle maker if needed and grease it.
5. Whisk eggs and sprinkle shredded cheddar cheese to them.
6. Mix all well and fill the mixture to the lower plate of the waffle maker.
7. Cook for at least 4 minutes to get the desired crunch.
8. Remove from the heat and divide into four pieces when cool down.
9. Mix all the vegetable, olives, coriander, and chaffles together and serve.

Nutrition:

- **Calories:** 391
- **Fat:** 21 g
- **Protein:** 14 g
- **Carbohydrates:** 10 g

Preparation Time: 25 minutes

Cooking Time: 7 minutes

Servings: 4

Ingredients:

- 2 eggs
- 1 cup Mozzarella cheese (shredded)
- 2 tbsp. cream cheese
- 1 tbsp. butter
- ½ cup onion:
- ½ cup tomato
- 1 tbsp. garlic powder
- Pepper: ¼ tsp.
- Basil: ½ tsp.
- ½ cup spinach
- 1 cup cauliflower florets:
- ¼ tsp. salt

Directions:

1. Take a pan, heat butter, add onion, and sauté for a minute.
2. Add tomatoes, spinach, and cauliflower and cook for 10 minutes.
3. Preheat your mini waffle iron if needed.
4. Mix all the ingredients mentioned above in a bowl with cauliflower and blend using a hand blender.
5. Grease your waffle iron lightly
6. Cook your mixture in the mini waffle iron for at least 4 minutes.
7. Serve hot with your favorite sauce
8. Make as many chaffles as your mixture and waffle maker allow.

Nutrition:

- **Calories:** 377
- **Fat:** 22 g
- **Protein:** 11 g
- **Carbohydrates:** 7 g

Preparation Time: 5 minutes

Cooking Time: 10 minutes

Servings: 2

Ingredients:

- 2 eggs
- 1½ cup Cheddar cheese
- 16 slices Deli jalapeno
- 1 cup spinach, chopped

Directions:

1. Boil water and add spinach and boil for 5 minutes.
2. Strain and drain to remove excess water.
3. Preheat a mini waffle maker if needed.
4. Beat eggs and add half cheddar cheese to them and mix well.
5. Shred some of the remaining cheddar cheese to the lower plate of the waffle maker.
6. Now pour the mixture into the shredded cheese and add in one spoon of spinach, and spread.
7. Add the cheese again on the top with around 4 slices of jalapeno and close the lid.
8. Cook for at least 4 minutes to get the desired crunch and serve hot.
9. Make as many chaffles as your mixture allows.

Nutrition:

- **Calories:** 339
- **Fat:** 28.2 g
- **Protein:** 19 g
- **Carbohydrates:** 26 g

Preparation Time: 5 minutes

Cooking Time: 7 minutes

Servings: 2

Ingredients:

- 1 egg
- ½ cup Mozzarella cheese (shredded)
- 2 chopped garlic cloves
- ½ cup pepper, finely chopped
- ½ cup onion, finely chopped
- Salt and pepper: to your taste

Directions:

1. Mix all the ingredients well together.
2. Pour a layer on a preheated waffle iron.
3. Cook the chaffle for around 5 minutes.
4. Make as many chaffles as your mixture and waffle maker allow.

Nutrition:

- **Calories:** 347
- **Fat:** 25 g
- **Protein:** 14 g
- **Carbohydrates:** 12 g

41. BASIL CHAFFLES

Preparation Time: 10 minutes

Cooking Time: 16 minutes

Servings: 3

Ingredients:

- 2 organic eggs, beaten
- ½ cup Mozzarella cheese, shredded
- 1 tbsp. Parmesan cheese, grated
- 1 tsp. dried basil, crushed
- Pinch salt

Directions:

1. Preheat a mini waffle iron and then grease it.
2. Incorporate all ingredients until well combined.
3. Place 1/3 of the mixture into preheated waffle iron and cook for about 3–4 minutes or until golden brown.
4. Repeat with the remaining mixture.
5. Serve warm.

Nutrition:

- **Calories:** 61
- **Fat:** 4.2 g
- **Protein:** 5.7 g
- **Carbohydrates:** 2 g

Preparation Time: 5 minutes

Cooking Time: 8 minutes

Servings: 2

Ingredients:

- 1 organic egg, beaten
- ½ cup Monterrey Jack cheese, shredded
- 1 tsp. coconut flour
- Pinch garlic powder

Directions:

1. Preheat a mini waffle iron and then grease it.
2. Incorporate all the ingredients until well combined.
3. Pour in half of the mixture into the prepared waffle iron and cook for about 3-4 minutes or until golden brown.
4. Repeat with the remaining mixture.
5. Serve warm.

Nutrition:

- **Calories:** 147
- **Fat:** 11.3 g
- **Protein:** 9 g
- **Carbohydrates:** 8 g

Preparation Time: 5 minutes

Cooking Time: 5 minutes

Servings: 1

Ingredients:

- 1 organic egg, beaten
- ¼ cup Cheddar cheese, shredded
- 2 tbsp. almond flour
- ½ tsp. organic baking powder
- ¼ tsp. garlic powder
- ¼ tsp. onion powder
- Pinch salt

Directions:

1. Preheat a waffle iron and then grease it.
2. Put all the ingredients and beat until well combined.
3. Place the mixture into preheated waffle iron and cook for about 3–5 minutes or until golden brown.
4. Serve warm.

Nutrition:

- **Calories**: 274
- **Fat**: 21.3 g
- **Protein**: 12.8 g
- **Carbohydrates**: 8 g

Preparation Time: 5 minutes

Cooking Time: 10 minutes

Servings: 2

Ingredients:

- ½ cup Mozzarella cheese, grated
- 1 medium organic egg, beaten
- 2 tbsp. almond flour
- ½ tsp. dried oregano, crushed
- ½ tsp. garlic powder
- Salt, to taste

Directions:

1. Preheat a mini waffle iron and then grease it.
2. Incorporate all ingredients until mix.
3. Pour in half of the mixture into prepared waffle iron and cook for about 4-5 minutes or until golden brown.
4. Repeat with the remaining mixture.
5. Serve warm.

Nutrition:

- **Calories**: 100
- **Fat**: 7.2 g
- **Protein**: 4.9 g
- **Carbohydrates**: 3 g

Preparation Time: 10 minutes

Cooking Time: 24 minutes

Servings: 6

Ingredients:

- ¾ cup coconut flour, sifted
- 1½ tsp. organic baking powder
- ½ tsp. dried ground sage
- 1/8 tsp. garlic powder
- 1/8 tsp. salt
- 1 organic egg
- 1 cup unsweetened coconut milk
- ¼ cup water
- 1½ tbsp. coconut oil, melted
- ½ cup cheddar cheese, shredded

Directions:

1. Preheat a waffle iron and then grease it.
2. In a bowl, add the flour, baking powder, sage, garlic powder, salt, and mix well.
3. Add the egg, coconut milk, water, and coconut oil and mix until a stiff mixture forms.
4. Add the cheese and gently stir to combine.
5. Divide the mixture into 6 portions.
6. Place 1 portion of the mixture into preheated waffle iron and cook for about 4 minutes or until golden brown.
7. Repeat with the remaining mixture.
8. Serve warm.

Nutrition:

- **Calories**: 147
- **Fat**: 13 g
- **Protein**: 4 g
- **Carbohydrates**: 5 g

Preparation Time: 5 minutes

Cooking Time: 8 minutes

Servings: 2

Ingredients:

- 1 organic egg, beaten
- ½ cup Cheddar cheese, shredded
- 1 tbsp. almond flour
- Pinch dried thyme, crushed
- Pinch dried rosemary, crushed

Directions:

1. Preheat a mini waffle iron and then grease it.
2. Mix all the ingredients.
3. Pour in half of the batter into prepared waffle iron and cook for about 3–4 minutes or until golden brown.
4. Repeat with the remaining mixture.
5. Serve warm.

Nutrition:

- **Calories:** 168
- **Fat:** 13.4 g
- **Protein:** 9.8 g
- **Carbohydrates:** 10 g

Preparation Time: 10 minutes

Cooking Time: 12 minutes

Servings: 4

Ingredients:

- 4 tbsp. almond flour
- 1 tbsp. coconut flour
- 1 tsp. mixed dried herbs
- ½ tsp. organic baking powder
- ¼ tsp. garlic powder
- ¼ tsp. onion powder
- ¼ cup cream cheese, softened
- 3 large organic eggs
- ½ cup Cheddar cheese, grated
- 1/3 cup Parmesan cheese, grated

Directions:

1. Preheat a waffle iron and then grease it.
2. In a bowl, mix together the flours, dried herbs, baking powder, seasoning, and mix well.
3. Whisk cream cheese and eggs and beat until well combined.
4. Add the flour mixture, cheddar, Parmesan cheese, and mix until well combined.
5. Place the desired amount of the mixture into preheated waffle iron and cook for about 2–3 minutes or until golden brown.
6. Repeat with the remaining mixture.
7. Serve warm.

Nutrition:

- **Calories**: 240
- **Fat**: 19 g
- **Protein**: 12.3 g
- **Carbohydrates**: 7 g

Preparation Time: 10 minutes

Cooking Time: 8 minutes

Servings: 2

Ingredients:

- 1 large organic egg, beaten
- ¼ cup Parmesan cheese, shredded
- ¼ cup Mozzarella cheese, shredded
- ½ tbsp. butter, melted
- 1 tsp. garlic herb blend seasoning
- Salt, to taste

Directions:

1. Preheat a mini waffle iron and then grease it.
2. Mix all the ingredients and beat it well.
3. Pour in half of the mixture into prepared waffle iron and cook for about 3-4 minutes or until golden brown.
4. Repeat with the remaining mixture.
5. Serve warm.

Nutrition:

- **Calories:** 115
- **Fat:** 8.8 g
- **Protein:** 8 g
- **Carbohydrates:** 6 g

Preparation Time: 5 minutes

Cooking Time: 8 minutes

Servings: 2

Ingredients:

- 1 organic egg, beaten
- ½ cup Cheddar cheese, shredded
- 1 tbsp. almond flour
- 1 tbsp. fresh rosemary, chopped

Directions:

1. Preheat a mini waffle iron and then grease it.
2. For chaffles: In a medium bowl, place all ingredients and with a fork and mix well.
3. Pour in half of the mixture into preheated waffle iron and cook for about 3–4 minutes or until golden brown.
4. Repeat with the remaining mixture.
5. Serve warm.

Nutrition:

- **Calories:** 173
- **Fat:** 13.7 g
- **Protein:** 9.9 g
- **Carbohydrates:** 7 g

Preparation Time: 15 minutes

Cooking Time: 24 minutes

Servings: 6

Ingredients:

- ½ cup ground flaxseed
- 2 organic eggs
- ½ cup goat cheddar cheese, grated
- 2-4 tbsp. plain Greek yogurt
- 1 tbsp. avocado oil
- ½ tsp. baking soda
- 1 tsp. fresh lemon juice
- 2 tbsp. fresh chives, minced
- 1 tbsp. fresh basil, minced
- ½ tbsp. fresh mint, minced
- ¼ tbsp. fresh thyme, minced
- ¼ tbsp. fresh oregano, minced

Directions:

1. Preheat a waffle iron and then grease it.
2. Incorporate all ingredients using a fork, mix until well combined.
3. Divide the mixture into 6 portions.
4. Place 1 portion of the mixture into preheated waffle iron and cook for about 4 minutes or until golden brown.
5. Repeat with the remaining mixture.
6. Serve warm.

Nutrition:

- **Calories**: 117
- **Fat**: 7.9 g
- **Protein**: 6.4 g
- **Carbohydrates**: 5 g

51. Minty Chaffle

Preparation Time: 15 minutes

Cooking Time: 7 minutes

Servings: 4

Ingredients:

- Egg: 2
- Cheddar cheese: 1 cup (shredded)
- Mint: ¼ cup chopped
- Onion: ½ cup chopped
- Cucumber: ½ cup chopped
- Tomato: ½ cup chopped
- Lettuce: ½ cup chopped
- Cabbage: ½ cup chopped
- Salt: ½ tsp.
- Black pepper: ¼ tsp.
- Fresh coriander: ½ cup chopped

Directions:

1. Preheat a mini waffle maker if needed and grease it.
2. Whisk eggs and sprinkle mint and shredded cheddar cheese to them.
3. Mix them all well, then fill the mixture to the lower plate of the waffle maker.
4. Cook for at least 4 minutes to get the desired crunch.
5. Remove from the heat and divide into four pieces when cool down.
6. Mix all the vegetable and seasoning and add the chaffles too and serve.

Nutrition:

- **Calories:** 461
- **Fat:** 22 g
- **Protein:** 11 g
- **Carbohydrates:** 6 g

Preparation Time: 15 minutes

Cooking Time: 8 minutes

Servings: 2

Ingredients:

- 1 packet tuna 2.6 oz. with no water
- ½ cup mozzarella cheese
- 1 egg
- Pinch salt

Directions:

1. Preheat the mini waffle maker
2. In a small bowl, add the egg and whip it up.
3. Add the tuna, cheese, and salt and mix well.
4. Optional step for an extra crispy crust: Add a tsp. of cheese to the mini waffle maker for about 30 seconds before adding the recipe mixture. This will allow the cheese to get crispy when the tuna chaffle is done cooking. I prefer this method!
5. Add ½ the mixture to the waffle maker and cook it for a minimum of 4 minutes.
6. Remove it and cook the last tuna chaffle for another 4 minutes.

Nutrition:

- **Calories**: 320
- **Carbohydrates**: 2.9 g
- **Protein**: 21.5 g
- **Fat**: 24.3 g

Preparation Time: 10 minutes

Cooking Time: 10 minutes

Ingredients:

- 2 chaffles
- 1 T Blueberry Compote
- 1 oz. Wisconsin Brie sliced thin
- 1 T Kerry gold butter

Chaffle Ingredients:

- 1 egg, beaten
- ¼ cup mozzarella shredded
- 1 tsp. Swerve confectioners
- 1 tbsp. cream cheese softened
- ¼ tsp. baking powder
- ½ tsp. vanilla extract

Blueberry Compote Ingredients:

- 1 cup blueberries washed
- Zest ½ lemon
- 1 tbsp. lemon juice freshly squeezed
- 1 tbsp. Swerve Confectioners
- 1/8 tsp. xanthan gum
- 2 tbsp. water

Directions:

1. Mix everything together.
2. Cook ½ batter for 2 ½–3 minutes in the mini waffle maker
3. Repeat.
4. Let cool slightly on a cooling rack.
5. Blueberry Compote Instructions:

6. Add everything except xanthan gum to a small saucepan. Bring to a boil, reduce heat and simmer for 5-10 minutes until it starts to thicken. Sprinkle with xanthan gum and stir well.

7. Remove from heat and let cool. Store in refrigerator until ready to use.

8. Grilled Cheese Instructions:

9. Heat butter in a small pan over medium heat. Place Brie slices on a Chaffle and top with a generous 1 T scoop of prepared blueberry compote.

10. Place sandwich in pan and grill, flipping once until waffle is golden and cheese has melted, about 2 minutes per side.

Nutrition:

- **Calories**: 320
- **Carbohydrates**: 2.9 g
- **Protein**: 21.5 g
- **Fat**: 24.3 g

54. BBQ Chicken Chaffle Waffle

Preparation Time: 3 minutes

Cooking Time: 8 minutes

Servings: 2

Ingredients:

- 1/3 cup cooked chicken diced
- ½ cup shredded cheddar cheese
- 1 tbsp. sugar-free BBQ sauce
- 1 egg
- 1 tbsp. almond flour

Directions:

1. Heat up your Dash mini waffle maker.
2. In a small bowl, mix the egg, almond flour, BBQ sauce, diced chicken, and Cheddar Cheese.
3. Add ½ of the batter into your mini waffle maker and cook for 4 minutes. If they are still a bit uncooked, leave it cooking for another 2 minutes. Then cook the rest of the batter to make a second chaffle.
4. Do not open the waffle maker before the 4-minute mark.
5. Enjoy alone or dip in BBQ Sauce or ranch dressing!

Nutrition:

- **Calories:** 320
- **Carbohydrates:** 2.9 g
- **Protein:** 21.5 g
- **Fat:** 24.3 g

Preparation Time: 2 minutes

Cooking Time: 8 minutes

Servings: 2

Ingredients:

- ¼ cup cooked diced chicken
- ¼ cup fresh broccoli chopped
- Shredded Cheddar cheese
- 1 egg
- ¼ tsp. garlic powder

Directions:

1. Heat up your Dash mini waffle maker.
2. In a small bowl, mix the egg, garlic powder, and cheddar cheese.
3. Add the broccoli and chicken and mix well.
4. Add ½ of the batter into your mini waffle maker and cook for 4 minutes. If they are still a bit uncooked, leave it cooking for another 2 minutes. Then cook the rest of the batter to make a second chaffle and then cook the third chaffle.
5. After cooking, remove from the pan and let sit for 2 minutes.
6. Dip in ranch dressing, sour cream, or enjoy alone.

Nutrition:

- **Calories:** 320
- **Carbohydrates:** 2.9 g
- **Protein:** 21.5 g
- **Fat:** 24.3 g

Preparation Time: 3 minutes

Cooking Time: 8 minutes

Servings: 2

Ingredients:

- 1/3 cup cooked diced chicken
- 1/3 cup cooked spinach chopped
- 1/3 cup marinated artichokes chopped
- 1/3 cup shredded mozzarella cheese
- 1 ounce softened cream cheese
- ¼ tsp. garlic powder
- 1 egg

Directions:

1. Heat up your Dash mini waffle maker.
2. In a small bowl, mix the egg, garlic powder, cream cheese, and Mozzarella Cheese.
3. Add the spinach, artichoke, and chicken and mix well.
4. Add 1/3 of the batter into your mini waffle maker and cook for 4 minutes. If they are still a bit uncooked, leave it cooking for another 2 minutes. Then cook the rest of the batter to make a second chaffle and then cook the third chaffle.
5. After cooking, remove from the pan and let sit for 2 minutes.
6. Dip in ranch dressing, sour cream, or enjoy alone.

Nutrition:

- **Calories:** 320
- **Carbohydrates:** 2.9 g
- **Protein:** 21.5 g
- **Fat:** 24.3 g

Preparation Time: 3 minutes

Cooking Time: 8 minutes

Servings: 2

Ingredients:

- 1 egg
- 1/3 cup cooked chicken diced
- 1 piece bacon cooked and crumbled
- 1/3 cup shredded cheddar jack cheese
- 1 tsp. powdered ranch dressing

Directions:

1. Heat up your Dash mini waffle maker.
2. In a small bowl, mix the egg, ranch dressing, and Monterey Jack Cheese.
3. Add the bacon and chicken and mix well.
4. Add half of the batter into your mini waffle maker and cook for 3-4 minutes. Then cook the rest of the batter to make a second chaffle.
5. Remove from the pan and let sit for 2 minutes.
6. Dip in ranch dressing, sour cream, or enjoy alone.

Nutrition:

- **Calories**: 220
- **Carbohydrates**: 2.9 g
- **Protein**: 21.5 g
- **Fat**: 24.3 g

Preparation Time: 10 minutes

Cooking Time: 5 minutes

Servings: 6

Ingredients:

- 1 Can Valley Fresh Organic Canned Chicken Breast (5 ounces)
- 2 tbsp. Red Hot Wing Sauce
- 2 oz. cream cheese softened
- 4 tbsp. Cheddar cheese shredded
- 2 tbsp. almond flour
- 1 tbsp. nutritional yeast
- ½ tsp. baking powder
- 1 egg yolk can use whole egg if no allergy
- 1 flax egg 1 T ground flaxseed, 3 T water
- ¼–½ cup extra cheese for the waffle iron

Directions:

1. Make flax egg and set it aside to rest.
2. Drain liquid from the canned chicken. Mix all the ingredients together. Sprinkle a little cheese on the waffle iron. Let it sit for a few seconds before adding 3 tbsp. of the chicken mixture—Cook for 5 minutes.
3. Don't open the waffle iron before the time is up, or you will have a mess. Remove and let cool before adding a drizzle of hot sauce and ranch dressing.

Nutrition:

- **Calories:** 320
- **Carbohydrates:** 2.9 g
- **Protein:** 21.5 g
- **Fat:** 24.3 g

Preparation Time: 5 minutes

Cooking Time: 10 minutes

Servings: 4

Ingredients:

Jamaican Jerk Chicken Filling:

- 1 pound organic ground chicken browned or roasted leftover chicken finely chopped
- 2 tbsp. Kerry gold butter
- ½ medium onion chopped
- 1 tsp. granulated garlic
- 1 tsp. dried thyme
- 1/8 tsp. black pepper
- 2 tsp. dried parsley
- 1 tsp. salt
- 2 tsp. Walker's Wood Jerk Seasoning Hot and Spicy jar type paste
- ½ cup chicken broth

Chaffle Ingredients:

- ½ cup mozzarella cheese
- 1 tbsp. butter melted
- 1 egg well beaten
- 2 tbsp. almond flour
- ¼ tsp. baking powder
- ¼ tsp. turmeric
- A pinch xanthan gum
- A pinch salt
- A pinch garlic powder
- A pinch onion powder

Directions:

1. In a medium saucepan, cook onion in the butter.
2. Add all spices and herbs. Sauté until fragrant.
3. Add chicken.
4. Stir in chicken broth.
5. Cook on low for 10 minutes.
6. Raise temperature to medium-high and reduce liquid until none is left in the bottom of the pan.

Nutrition:

- **Calories**: 320
- **Carbohydrates**: 2.9 g
- **Protein**: 21.5 g
- **Fat**: 24.3 g

Preparation Time: 15 minutes

Cooking Time: 15 minutes

Servings: 1

Ingredient

- Classic Chaffle Recipe

Japanese Toppings Ingredients:

- 1 whole avocado, ripe
- 5 slices pickled ginger
- 1 tbsp. gluten-free soy sauce
- 1/3 cup edamame
- ¼ cup Japanese pickled vegetables
- ½ pound sushi-grade salmon, sliced
- ¼ tsp. wasabi

Directions:

1. Cut the salmon and avocado into thin slices. Set aside.
2. If the edamame is frozen, boil it in a pot of water until done. Set aside.
3. Follow the Classic Chaffle recipe.
4. Once the chaffles are done, pour a tbsp. of soy sauce onto the chaffle and then layer the salmon, avocado, edamame, pickled ginger, pickled vegetables, and wasabi.

Nutrition:

- **Calories**: 320
- **Carbohydrates**: 2.9 g
- **Protein**: 21.5 g
- **Fat**: 24.3 g

Preparation Time: 15 minutes

Cooking Time: 15 minutes

Servings: 1

Ingredients:

- Classic Chaffle Recipe

Nacho Ingredients:

- Taco Meat recipe
- 1 whole avocado, ripe
- ½ cup sour cream
- ½ cup cheddar cheese, shredded
- ½ an onion
- 1 handful cilantro, chopped
- 1 lime, cut into wedges
- Hot sauce your choice

Directions:

1. Dice the cilantro, lettuce, onions, and limes.
2. Shred the cheese in a bowl. Melt if desired.
3. Follow instructions for the Taco Meat recipe.
4. Follow the Classic Chaffle recipe.
5. Once the chaffles are done, rip them into triangles.
6. Spread the chaffle triangles onto a plate and layer on the sour cream, meat, avocado, onions, cilantro, cheese, and lime.
7. Enjoy!

Nutrition:

- **Calories:** 320
- **Carbohydrates:** 2.9 g
- **Protein:** 21.5 g
- **Fat:** 24.3 g

62. Mozzarella Panini

Preparation Time: 15 minutes

Cooking Time: 15 minutes

Servings: 1

Ingredients:

- Classic Chaffle Recipe

Sandwich Filling Ingredients:

- 1 ounce mozzarella, thinly sliced
- 1 heirloom tomato, thinly sliced
- ¼ cup pesto
- 2 fresh basil leaves

Directions:

1. Follow the Classic Chaffle recipe.
2. Once the chaffles are done, lay two side by side.
3. Spread the pesto on one, then layer the mozzarella cheese and tomatoes and sandwich together.

Nutrition:

- **Calories:** 1 320
- **Carbohydrates:** 2.9 g
- **Protein:** 21.5 g
- **Fat:** 24.3 g

63. LOX CHAFFLE

Preparation Time: 15 minutes

Cooking Time: 15 minutes

Servings: 1

Ingredients:

- Classic Chaffle Recipe or Sweet Chaffle Recipe
- 2 tbsp. Everything Bagel Seasoning

Filling Ingredients:

- 1 ounce cream cheese
- 1 beefsteak tomato, thinly sliced
- 4-6 ounces salmon gravlax
- 1 small shallot, thinly sliced
- capers
- 1 tbsp. fresh dill

Directions:

1. Slice the tomato and the shallots.
2. Follow the Classic Chaffle recipe and add bagel seasoning.
3. Once the chaffles are done, sprinkle more everything bagel seasoning onto the tops of both chaffles.
4. Lay two chaffles side by side and layer on the cream cheese, salmon, and shallots.
5. Sprinkle dill and capers and sandwich the two chaffles together.
6. Enjoy!

Nutrition:

- **Calories:** 320
- **Carbohydrates:** 2.9 g
- **Protein:** 21.5 g
- **Fat:** 24.3 g

Preparation Time: 15 minutes

Cooking Time: 15 minutes

Servings: 1

Ingredients:

- Classic Chaffle Recipe

Cuban **Ingredients:**

- ¼ pound ham, cooked and sliced
- ¼ pound pork, roasted and sliced
- ¼-pound Swiss cheese, thinly sliced
- 3 dill pickles, sliced in half

Directions:

1. Follow the Classic Chaffle recipe.
2. Take two chaffles and lay side by side.
3. Lay on the meat, cheese, and pickles.
4. Sandwich the two chaffles together.
5. Put the sandwich in a toaster oven if you want it hot.
6. Heat for 5 minutes or until cheese is melted.

Nutrition:

- **Calories**: 329
- **Carbohydrates**: 2 g
- **Protein**: 25 g
- **Fat**: 24.3 g

Preparation Time: 10 minutes

Cooking Time: 5 minutes

Servings: 2

Ingredients:

- ½ cup shredded mozzarella cheese
- 1 whole egg, beaten
- ¼ cup grated Parmesan cheese
- 1 tsp. Italian Seasoning
- ¼ tsp. garlic powder

Directions:

1. Start preheating your waffle maker, and let's start preparing the batter.
2. Add in all the ingredients, except for the mozzarella cheese, to a bowl and whisk. Add in the cheese and mix until well combined.
3. Spray your waffle plates with nonstick spray and add half the batter to the center. Close the lid and cook for 3–5 minutes, depending on how crispy you want.
4. Serve with a drizzle of olive oil, grated Parmesan cheese, and fresh chopped parsley or basil.

Nutrition:

- **Calories**: 320
- **Carbohydrates**: 2.9 g
- **Protein**: 21.5 g
- **Fat**: 24.3 g

Preparation Time: 10 minutes

Cooking Time: 5 minutes

Servings: 2

Ingredients:

- 1 egg
- 2 tsp. cream cheese room temp
- 1 tsp. powdered sweetener swerve or monk fruit
- ½ tsp. baking powder
- ½ tsp. lime zest
- ¼ cup almond flour
- ½ tsp. lime extract or 1 tsp. fresh-squeezed lime juice
- Pinch salt

Cream Cheese Lime Frosting:

- 4 oz. cream cheese softened
- 4 tbsp. butter
- 2 tsp. powdered sweetener swerve or monk fruit
- 1 tsp. lime extract
- ½ tsp. lime zest

Directions:

1. Preheat the mini waffle iron.
2. In a blender, add all the chaffle ingredients and blend on high until the mixture is smooth and creamy.
3. Cook each chaffle for about 3 to 4 minutes until they are golden brown.
4. While the chaffles are cooking, prepare the frosting.
5. In a small bowl, combine all the ingredients for the frosting and mix until smooth.
6. Allow the chaffles to cool completely before frosting them.

Nutrition:

- **Calories:** 348
- **Carbohydrates:** 2.9 g
- **Protein:** 26 g
- **Fat:** 21 g

Preparation Time: 10 minutes

Cooking Time: 15 minutes

Servings: 2

Ingredients:

- 1 cup cheese choice
- 2 eggs, whisked
- 1 large jicama root
- ½ medium onion, minced
- Salt and pepper
- 2 garlic cloves, pressed

Directions:

1. Peel jicama and shred in food processor
2. In a large colander, place the shredded jicama, and sprinkle with 1–2 tsp. of salt. Mix well and allow to drain.
3. Squeeze out as much liquid as possible.
4. Microwave for 5–8 minutes
5. Mix all ingredients together
6. Sprinkle a little cheese on the waffle iron, then add 1/3 of the mixture, and sprinkle a little more cheese on top of the mixture.
7. Cook for 5 minutes. Flip and cook 2 more.
8. Top with a dollop of sour cream, bacon pieces, cheese, and chives.

Nutrition:

- **Calories**: 320
- **Carbohydrates**: 2.9 g
- **Protein**: 21.5 g
- **Fat**: 24.3 g

Preparation Time: 10 minutes

Cooking Time: 5 minutes

Servings: 2

Ingredients:

- 1 egg
- 3/4 cup shredded Mozzarella
- 1 sausage patty
- 1 slice American cheese
- 1 tbsp. sugar-free flavored maple syrup
- 1 tbsp. Swerve or Monk fruit (or any sugar replacement of choice)

Directions:

1. Preheat your Mini Waffle Maker
2. Beat the egg into a small mixing bowl,
3. Add shredded Mozzarella, Swerve/Monk fruit, Maple Syrup and mix until well combined.
4. Place ~2 tbsp. of the resulting egg mix onto the Dash Mini Waffle Maker, close lid, and cook for 3–4 minutes. Repeat for as many waffles as you are making.
5. Meanwhile, follow cooking instructions for sausage patty and place cheese onto patty while still warm to melt.
6. Assemble Chaffle Griddle and enjoy!

Nutrition:

- **Calories**: 320
- **Carbohydrates**: 2.9 g
- **Protein**: 21.5 g
- **Fat**: 24.3 g

Preparation Time: 10 minutes

Cooking Time: 5 minutes

Servings: 2

Ingredients:

- 1 egg
- 1/3 cup cheddar
- ¼ tsp. baking powder
- ½ tsp. ground flaxseed
- Shredded parmesan cheese on top and bottom.

Directions:

1. Mix the ingredients together and cook in a mini waffle iron for 4-5 minutes until crispy.
2. Once cool, enjoy your light and crisp Keto waffle.
3. You can experiment with seasonings to the initial mixture depending on the mood of your taste buds.

Nutrition:

- **Calories:** 327
- **Carbohydrates:** 21.7 g
- **Protein:** 20.3 g
- **Fat:** 24.3 g

Preparation Time: 10 minutes

Cooking Time: 5 minutes

Servings: 2

Ingredients:

- 1 large egg
- ½ cup shredded cheese
- Thick-cut bacon
- Fried egg
- Sliced cheese

Directions:

1. Preheat your waffle maker.
2. In a small mixing bowl, mix together egg and shredded cheese. Stir until well combined.
3. Pour one-half of the waffle batter into the waffle maker. Cook for 3–4 minutes or until golden brown. Repeat with the second half of the batter.
4. In a large pan over medium heat, cook the bacon until crispy.
5. In the same skillet, in 1 tbsp. of reserved bacon drippings, fry the egg over medium heat. Cook until the desired doneness.
6. Assemble the sandwich, and enjoy!

Nutrition:

- **Calories:** 320
- **Carbohydrates:** 2.9 g
- **Protein:** 21.5 g
- **Fat:** 24.3 g

71. RICH CREAMY CHAFFLES

Preparation Time: 5 minutes

Cooking Time: 5 minutes

Servings: 4

Ingredients:

- 1 egg
- ½ cup mozzarella cheese, shredded
- Oil grease
- Heavy crème
- Salt & pepper to taste

Directions:

1. Heat the waffle maker. Take a bowl, add an egg or mozzarella cheese and whisk all together. Add some salt or pepper as per taste and mix all together. Spray the oil to grease the waffle maker. Now pour the mixture into the maker and cook for 4 minutes or until golden brown. Repeat the process for the whole batter. Serve the chaffle with a heavy crème layer.

Nutrition:

- **Calories:** 344
- **Carbohydrates:** 20 g
- **Protein:** 26 g
- **Fat:** 23 g

Chapter 7.

MEDIUM DIFFICULTY CHAFFLE RECIPES

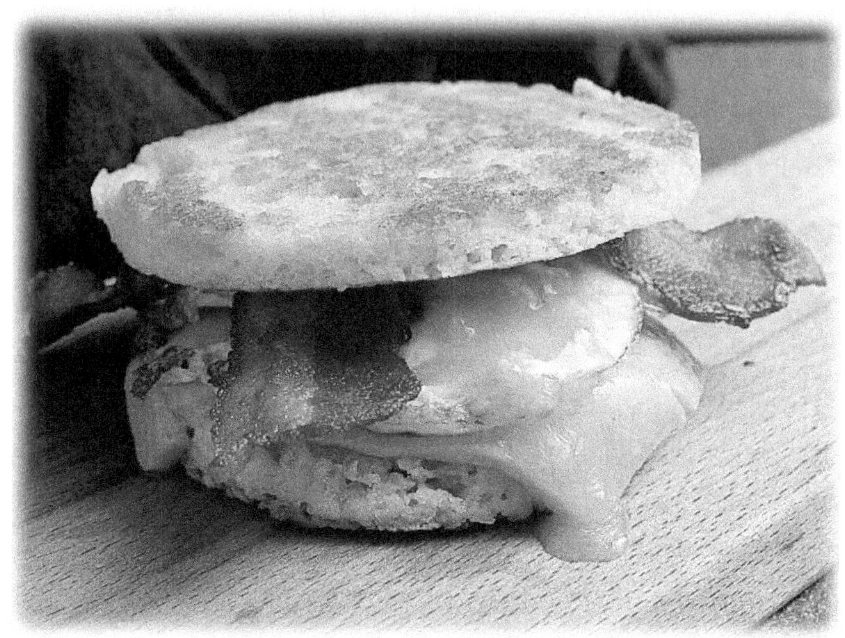

72. BLT CHAFFLE SANDWICH

Preparation Time: 5 minutes

Cooking Time: 5 minutes

Servings: 2

Ingredients:

For Chaffle:

- ½ cup, shredded mozzarella
- 1 egg
- 1 tbsp. green onion, chopped
- ½ tsp. Seasoning (Italian)

For Sandwich:

- Pre-cooked bacon
- Lettuce

- Tomato, in slices
- 1 tbsp. mayo

Directions:

1. Heat up the mini-waffle maker.
2. Whip the egg in a little bowl.
3. Add the cheese, seasonings, and onion to blend. Mix until it's fully set in.
4. In the mini waffle maker, place half the batter and cook for 4 minutes.
5. If you want a crunchy crust, apply a tsp. of grated cheese to the mini waffle iron before adding the batter for 30 seconds. Extra cheese will create the best crust on the outside.
6. Following the completion of the first chaffle, add the rest batter to the waffle maker and cook for 4 minutes.
7. Fill your sandwich with mayo, Bacon, lettuce, and tomato.

Nutrition:

- **Calories**: 183
- **Fat**: 13.9 g
- **Protein**: 10.8 g
- **Carbohydrates**: 8 g

Preparation Time: 8 minutes

Cooking Time: 7 minutes

Servings: 2

Ingredients:

- 1 egg, should be large
- ½ cup crushed cheddar, mozzarella, or any grated cheese
- ¼ cup almond flour.
- ¼ tsp. gluten-free baking powder
- 2 ham slices
- 57 g - 2 slices cheese
- 4 - 60 g tomato slices
- 15 g - 2 small leaves lettuce
- Optional: 1 or 2 tbsp. cream cheese, butter, or mayonnaise.

Directions:

1. Start making the chaffles as per the directions. Either you can create 2 standard chaffles, or 3 thinner ones.
2. Let the chaffles all cool down. They will be soft when hot but will crisp when getting colder.
3. Fill with ham, cheese, lettuce, and tomato croutons. Optionally, before filling, you can add 1 to 2 spoonsful of cream cheese and spread it over the chaffles.
4. Immediately enjoy or place the chaffles in a sealed container for up to 3 days at room temperature or in the refrigerator for up to a week. Freeze for up to 3 months, for longer storage. The jar would maintain the soft texture, but if you want crispy, you should leave them untouched.

Nutrition:

- **Calories:** 733
- **Fat:** 57.1 g
- **Protein:** 45.8 g
- **Carbohydrates:** 38 g

74. KETO BREAKFAST CHAFFLE SANDWICH

Preparation Time: 5 minutes

Cooking Time: 7 minutes

Servings: 2

Ingredients:

- 1 Large egg
- ½ shredded cheese (cheddar)
- 2 tsp. mayonnaise
- 1–2 pcs bacon
- 1 egg

Directions:

1. Heat up the mini waffle iron.
2. Add the shredded cheese and the egg in a little bowl, whereas the waffle iron is heating.
3. Pour half the batter into the waffle maker and cook 3–4 minutes or until done.
4. Cook the bacon in a small saucepan until crispy nicely browned, then set aside.
5. Cook the egg to ideal doneness using the same tiny saucepan, add sea salt and pepper to fit.
6. Put in the mayonnaise, bacon, and egg to the chaffle.

Nutrition:

- **Calories:** 346.6
- **Fat:** 27.9 g
- **Protein:** 22.5 g
- **Carbohydrates:** 18 g

Preparation Time: 8 minutes

Cooking Time: 7 minutes

Servings: 2

Ingredients:

Cajun Aromatized Chaffle:

- 4 eggs, should be large
- 2 cups shredded mozzarella part-skim cheese
- 1 tsp. Seasoning Cajun

Filling for Sandwich:

- 1-pound fresh shrimp peeled and deveined
- 1 tbsp. bacon (or avocado) grease
- 4 slices bacon cooked
- 1 large sliced avocado
- ¼ cup red onion, thinly sliced
- 1 dish bacon scallion cream cheese spread optional
- 1 tsp. Seasoning (Cajun)

Directions:

1. Whisk the eggs together. Add 2 cups of mozzarella cheese with low moisture and 1 tsp. of Cajun seasoning. Put ¼ cup of cheese and a mixture of eggs over a mini waffle pan. Cook until the chaffle is browned. Repeat the process with the left egg and cheese batter.
2. Add shrimp and combine it in a large bowl, with the remaining 1 tsp. of Cajun seasoning. Garnish with salt and pepper. Fried in a pan over medium-high heat with bacon grease until the shrimp is translucent. Lift the fried shrimp and put aside. Let cool if desired.
3. Place bacon scallion cream cheese over a side of a chaffle to create the Chaffle Sandwich: cover the top of the chaffle with shrimp, bacon, avocado and red onion. Cover with one more chaffle. Serve as you wish.

Nutrition:

- **Calories**: 488
- **Fat**: 32.2 g
- **Protein**: 47.59 g
- **Carbohydrates**: 33 g

Preparation Time: 4 minutes

Cooking Time: 7 minutes

Servings: 2

Ingredients:

For wonder-bread chaffle:

- 2 eggs white
- 2 tbsp. almond flour
- 1 tbsp. mayonnaise
- 1 tsp. water
- ¼ tsp. baking powder
- 1 pinch salt

For sandwich elements:

- 2 tbsp. mayonnaise
- 1-piece deli ham
- 1 slice deli turkey
- 1 slice cheese cheddar
- 1 tomato slice
- 1 leaf green leaf lettuce

Directions:

1. Preheat the maker. Mix all the ingredients of the wonder-bread chaffle in a tiny bowl. White bread chaffle components combined together in a large bowl.
2. Place ½ the batter into the waffle maker and cook for about 3 to 5 minutes until finished.
3. Wonder-bread chaffle batter in a little waffle-maker.
4. Remove the waffle when cooking has been completed. Repeat for the batter remaining.
5. Made keto sandwich bread in a waffle maker.
6. Place mayonnaise on one side of each bread chaffle sandwich. Place in green leaf, tomato, and cold cuts.

Nutrition:

- **Calories:** 208
- **Fat:** 17.4 g
- **Protein:** 10.3 g
- **Carbohydrates:** 8 g

Preparation Time: 6 minutes

Cooking Time: 7 minutes

Servings: 2

Ingredients:

- 1 egg
- ½ cup mozzarella cheese
- 2 tbsp. flour (almond)
- 2 tbsp. low carbohydrate thousand island dressing
- ¼ tsp. baking powder
- ¼ tsp. seeds caraway
- 2 corned beef slices
- 1 Swiss cheese slice
- 2 tbsp. sauerkraut

Directions:

1. Set the temperature to the mid-high heat of the waffle maker.
2. In a bowl, mix together the egg, mozzarella, almond flour, a tbsp. of low carb dressing seeds of caraway as well as baking powder.
3. Place the chaffle batter into the waffle maker center. Shut the waffle machine and let it be cooked for 5 to 7 minutes or till lightly browned and crisp is perfect. If a mini waffle maker is used, just spill half the mixture over the waffle machine. Two chaffles (mini) will be produced from this recipe.
4. Take chaffle out from the waffle machine. If you are using a mini waffle machine, repeat for the residual batter.
5. Place the corned beef on a sheet of parchment, and cover with a Swiss cheese slice. Heat for 20 to 30 sec in the oven before the cheese begins to melt. Take off from the microwave. Place on each chaffle the remaining tbsp. of low carbohydrate thousand island sauces spread the Swiss cheese and hot corned beef, and finish with sauerkraut as well as other chaffle.

Nutrition:

- **Calories:** 605
- **Fat:** 43.8 g
- **Protein:** 45.1 g
- **Carbohydrates:** 34 g

Preparation Time: 15 minutes

Cooking Time: 7 minutes

Servings: 2

Ingredients:

- 10 eggs
- 1 ½ cups cheddar cheese, shredded
- 2 center-cut slices bacon, cooked and crumbled
- ½ tsp. ground pepper
- 2 small, sliced avocados
- 2 little tomatoes, in slices
- 4 large lettuce leaves, torn into 3 "parts

Directions:

1. In a large bowl, whisk the eggs until smooth. Stir in cheese and chopped bacon and pepper.
2. Preheat a 7-inch (not Belgian) round waffle iron; top it with cooking spray. Pour approximately 2/3 cup of the beaten egg into the waffle iron. Cook 4 to 5 minutes till the eggs are set and light golden brown. Repeat with cooking spray and the residual mixture of eggs (making a total of 4 chaffles).
3. Split each of the chaffles into pieces. Top half of the quarters even with slices of avocado, tomato slices, and lettuce. Also, top the remaining quarters of the chaffle.

Nutrition:

- **Calories:** 259
- **Fat:** 20.1 g
- **Protein:** 14 g
- **Carbohydrates:** 12 g

Preparation Time: 5 minutes

Cooking Time: 7 minutes

Servings: 2

Ingredients:

- ½ cup grated mozzarella
- 1 medium beaten egg
- 2 tbsp. almond flour

Filling:

- 2 slices turkey
- 3 Slices Brie
- 2 tbsp. chia cranberry jam

Directions:

1. Turn your waffle maker on and grease it gently.
2. Add the egg, mozzarella, and almond flour to a bowl. Combine until mixed.
3. Spoon the mixture into the waffle maker. If you want a small waffle maker, spoon half the batter in at a time).
4. Close the lid and cook until golden and firm for 5 minutes.
5. Use tongs to remove the cooked waffles and set them aside.
6. Place the turkey, brie, and cranberry on a cutting board and layer on the chaffle. Put the layers together with your choice.
7. Place on top of the other chaffle and slice in half.
8. If you just want a warm sandwich, then heat it up for 20 seconds in the microwave.

Nutrition:

- Calories: 537
- **Fat:** 36 g
- **Protein:** 44 g
- **Carbohydrates:** 31 g

Preparation Time: 5 minutes

Cooking Time: 7 minutes

Servings: 2

Ingredients:

- 1 large egg
- ½ cup mozzarella
- 1 tbsp. standard, gluten-free, almond or coconut flour
- ½ tsp. baking powder
- 1 pinch salt

Directions:

1. Coat nonstick cooking spray on the interior of a waffle maker. Preheat the waffle maker.
2. Beat the egg in a little mixing bowl or cup. Mix the flour, baking powder, salt and combine properly.
3. Stir in the scrambled cheese.
4. Put the batter into the waffle iron. When using a mini-waffle machine, simply add in half of the mix.
5. Lower with the cover. If the waffle maker has indicated the waffle is finished, raise the cover and transfer the waffle gently to a cooling rack. Use tongs to protect the fingertips from burning.
6. Repeat this step until the amount of the chaffles you want is reached.

Nutrition:

- Calories: 269
- **Fat:** 17 g
- **Protein:** 20 g
- **Carbohydrates:** 11 g

Preparation Time: 5 minutes

Cooking Time: 7 minutes

Servings: 2

Ingredients:

- 10 tbsp. parmesan shredded cheese
- 1 cup mozzarella shredded
- 2 slices bacon (chopped)
- ¼ tsp. dry oregano
- 1 heaping tbsp. birch benders pancake mix
- 2 eggs
- Mayo
- 2 tiny or 1 large, thinly cut tomato
- Salt and pepper to fit

Directions:

1. Put the egg, oregano, mozzarella cheese pancake mixture and salt and pepper into a food processor. Pulse blend until complete. Should just take a few steps.
2. Add bacon and pulse in the mixture until bacon is uniformly dispersed.
3. Put 1 tbsp. of parmesan on the waffle maker bottom. 1 Heaping waffle mixture spoonful and 1 tbsp. parmesan on top. Cover the waffle maker and finish cooking till golden brown. Repeat until the entire mix is used. It can yield about five mini waffles.
4. Apply mayo on the waffle side. Add sliced tomato, salt and pepper to taste. Attach 2nd waffle to the end.

Nutrition:

- **Calories:** 320
- **Fat:** 24 g
- **Protein:** 21 g
- **Carbohydrates:** 16 g

Preparation Time: 5 minutes

Cooking Time: 7 minutes

Servings: 2

Ingredients:

- 2 batches chaffle simple recipe
- 2 strips sugar-free bacon
- 2 oz. free sugar sliced deli turkey
- 2 oz. sugar-free sliced deli ham
- 1 slice cheese (cheddar)
- 1 tomato slice
- 3 lettuce leaves
- 1 tbsp. mayonnaise free sugar

Directions:

1. Cook the chaffles and put them aside, as instructed. Cover to keep warm.
2. Cook the Bacon using your chosen (oven/microwave/stovetop) cooking process. By putting those in the microwave, sealed, keep it basic for around 2–3 minutes (based on how crispy you want it and the brand). When cooked, move to a lined sheet of paper towel.
3. Make your sandwich, start the club sandwich with one chaffle, and complete with the tomato and the lettuce. Add the other chaffle and the cheese, ham, turkey, and bacon on top. Smear the final chaffle with mayo, then put it on top of the sandwich.
4. Enjoy it right away.

Nutrition:

- **Calories:** 178
- **Fat:** 8.6 g
- **Protein:** 6.6 g
- **Carbohydrates:** 8 g

Preparation Time: 5 minutes

Cooking Time: 7 minutes

Servings: 2

Ingredients:

Waffle:

- ¾ cup (75 g) shredded cheese (your choice)
- 1 medium-sized egg
- 1 tsp. husk psyllium
- salt/pepper
- Hot sauce (Optional)

Sandwich:

- 4 bacon strips
- 4 ham slices
- 4 prosciutto slices
- 5–6 salami slices
- 5–6 small pepperoni slices
- Mustard
- Mayonnaise

Directions:

1. Whisk the egg, cheese, salt, pepper, psyllium husk together in a bowl, and additional hot sauce.
2. Keep the waffle maker to heat until the batter is uniformly poured into the waffle pan.
3. Cook 2–3 minutes or more based on how crispy you like it to be.
4. Carry it out and eat the sandwich as is or top with delicious ingredients, fat-filled dinner.

Nutrition:

- **Calories:** 458
- **Fat:** 33.4 g
- **Protein:** 26.7 g
- **Carbohydrates:** 38 g

Preparation Time: 15 minutes

Cooking Time: 7 minutes

Servings: 2

Ingredients:

- 1 pork butt—bone-in
- 8 tbsp. barbecue sauce - sugar-free
- 1 packet coleslaw mix or chopped cabbage
- 1 cup mayo
- 2 tbsp. heavy cream
- 1 tsp. creole mustard (any mustard you want, etc.)
- 1 tbsp. erythritol
- 1 tsp. (Optional) pepper
- 1 tsp. garlic powder
- 1 tsp. black chili pepper
- 1 tsp. salt

Directions:

1. It begins with "scoring" the roast's fat side. The scoring helps the seasoning to enter the fat and add this to another flavor.
2. Use cooking oils, butter, mustard, Worcestershire sauce, or any other chosen "wet" ingredient to add a slight element of moisture to enable the seasonings or rub to stick better to the meat.
3. Cover the whole piece of meat absolutely with your favorite rub and let it sit for around 15-20 minutes until burning your Pit Barrel.
4. Place the fat side of the pork butt on the grill so that the meat is covered, and the fat becomes crisper if you cut the pork into pieces for taste and texture pieces. Smoke exposed inside until it hits 165 degrees. Put it in a foil tray, cover it and position it again in the cooker once 205 degrees is achieved.
5. Take out the pan and let it cool. To remove the fat from the liquids, dump any liquid from the pan into another dish. Then place the juices back in the pan and start cutting the pork roast into medium-sized chunks and scraping any big fat or tendon pieces.

6. Spray the same rub you cooked with over the pulled bits to provide a few extra spices, and spray it with the cooking sauces.

7. Combine all coleslaw dressing components and check taste for further changes to the seasoning. Toss the coleslaw (or cabbage mix) with the sauce. Coleslaw may appear thicker to begin with but will change for 1 hour while resting in the fridge.

8. Heat waffle iron for waffles. Drop one slice of cheese onto the waffle iron or scatter grated mozzarella cheese to cover the waffle maker's rim. Place ½ of a deviled egg over the cheese, which might melt. Place segmented cheese slice or cover with grated cheese and cover waffle iron. If you like it to be crunchier, let it steam for 3 minutes (until sides crisp) or more. When it cools, it can become crunchier, so check first to see what consistency you want and then change the period accordingly.

9. Place the chaffle sandwich together or eat in a bowl if you like to skip the chaffles.

10. Use this remaining pulled pork at lunch for the next two days.

Nutrition:

- **Calories**: 100
- **Fat**: 4.8 g
- **Protein**: 8.8 g
- **Carbohydrates**: 4.8 g

Preparation Time: 5 minutes

Cooking Time: 7 minutes

Servings: 2

Ingredients:

- 2 large raw eggs
- 2 tbsp. coconut flour
- 2 tbsp. mayo
- ½ tsp. baking powder
- 1 tsp. absolute substitute icing sugar by swerve
- 1 x 2 patties brown banquet, and serve patties
- ¾ ounces—2 slice American cheese slices

Directions:

1. At medium-high temperature, preheat the waffle iron. In a big mixing dish, add two whites, coconut flour, mayo, baking powder, and whisk.
2. Whisk well. Let the batter stay for around 1 minute to thicken.
3. Spray waffle iron with nonstick spray high heat grill. Put into hot waffle iron and cook as directed by iron. Take away waffles from the iron. Slice the chaffle in half.
4. Meanwhile, use a nonstick cooking spray with a 4 oz. ramekin. Add one egg and gently scramble it with a fork. Place completely cooked sausage patty in the middle and microwave for around 1 minute on 60 percent power before the egg is cooked through.
5. Put egg and sausage with a slice of American cheese on a quarter of the chaffle. Repeat on the other sandwich with the cooking of another egg and sausage. Right away, enjoy or freeze in plastic wrap.

Nutrition:

- **Calories**: 433
- **Fat**: 28.4 g
- **Protein**: 17.6 g
- **Carbohydrates**: 14 g

Preparation Time: 15 minutes

Cooking Time: 7 minutes

Servings: 2

Ingredients:

- 3-4 bacon pieces
- 1 egg
- ½ cup mozzarella
- 1 tsp. flour almonds
- 1 tsp. all Bagel Seasoning (or preferably a sprinkle salt, garlic, onion powder)
- 2 lettuce slices
- 1 sliced tomato
- 1 avocado slice
- 1 tbsp. mayonnaise

Directions:

For Bacon:

1. Start with a cold saucepan. Put the bacon in the pan and turn on the heat to a minimum. At minimum temperature, bacon cooks better. When the bacon warms up a little bit and loses more of its fat, it begins curling up gently. You can then use tongs to rotate the bacon and start cooking on the other side. Then proceed to turn consistently until all sides of the bacon are fried, around 10 minutes for thin or up to 15 minutes for thicker sliced bacon.

For Sandwich:

1. Plugin, the Mini Waffle maker, to preheat.
2. Crack the egg into a little bowl to create the chaffle and blend along with ½ cup mozzarella, almond flour, and all bagel seasoning. This blend produces 2 chaffles.
3. Pour ½ of the mix into the preheated chaffle maker and permit 3–4 minutes of cooking (depending on how crispy you like your chaffles).
4. When cooking your first chaffle, prepare the tomato and avocado by cutting one slice of each.
5. Pick up the chaffle and repeat for 3–4 minutes, adding the other half of the blend into the chaffle machine. When done, unplug the Waffle Machine.

6. In the chaffle, add your fried bacon, then finish with lettuce, tomato, avocado, and mayo.

7. Put 2 toothpicks in the chaffle to tie them together and slice them in half. Your chaffle BLT avocado is ready to serve now.

Nutrition:

- **Calories**: 208
- **Fat**: 19.4 g
- **Protein**: 20.3 g
- **Carbohydrates**: 12 g

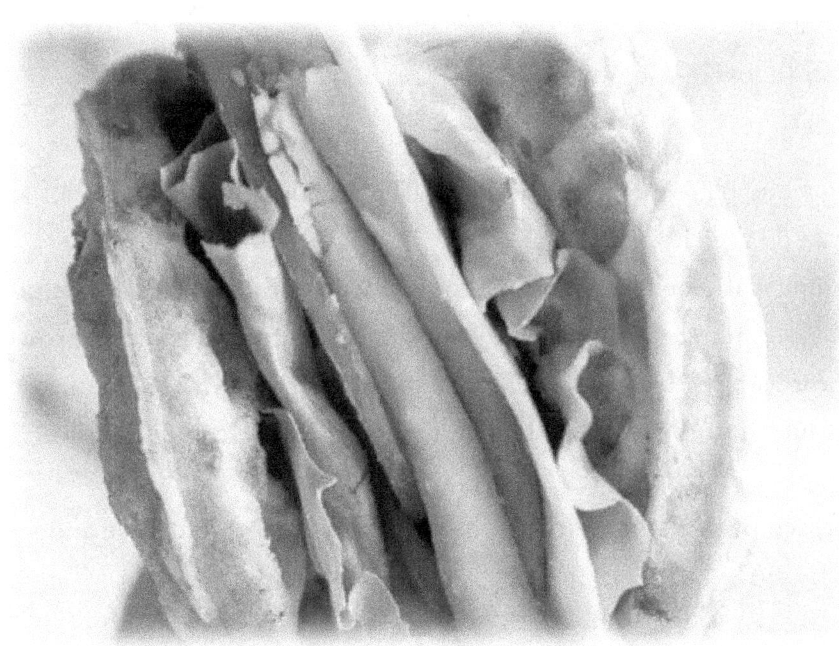

Preparation Time: 5 minutes

Cooking Time: 7 minutes

Servings: 2

Ingredients:

- 4 ounces roasted beef
- 2 eggs (egg whites only)
- 2 tbsp. almond flour
- 1 tbsp. sour cream
- 1-½ cup mozzarella
- ½ cup beef broth low in sodium

Directions:

1. Whip the egg white till foamy to make the chaffle. Include the almond flour and sour cream and mix properly. Add the cheese in.
2. Heat up the mini waffle maker according to instructions from the manufacturer. When heated and cook for 7–10 minutes, add half the batter once the chaffle is nicely browned and readily releases. Repeat with the batter left behind.
3. In the meanwhile, heat the beef broth in a tiny pot or pan. Heat up the sliced beef, don't overcook it!
4. Put the processed beef on the chaffle to be assembled, top with cheese and serve sideways with the available broth.

Nutrition:

- **Calories:** 444
- **Fat:** 26 g
- **Protein:** 45 g
- **Carbohydrates:** 14 g

Preparation Time: 15 minutes

Cooking Time: 7 minutes

Servings: 2

Ingredients:

- 1 egg
- 3/4 cup almond flour
- ½ tsp. baking powder
- 1/8 t salt
- 2 tbsp. melted butter
- ¼ cup mozzarella shredded cheese
- ¼ cup sour cream

Directions:

1. Mix together the ingredients and place the batter into a mini waffle iron to produce a batch of chaffles
2. Tuna Sandwich: Take two chaffles and bring them together to make a sandwich with your St. Jude tuna salad. Choose your unique flavor of St. Jude tuna: blend with a little bit of olive oil and pepper. Add pepperoncini, tomatoes, red onion, red peppers, and all other preferred toppings

Nutrition:

- **Calories**: 100
- **Fat**: 3.7 g
- **Protein**: 9.6 g
- **Carbohydrates**: 8 g

Preparation Time: 5 minutes

Cooking Time: 7 minutes

Servings: 2

Ingredients:

- 1 large egg
- 1 tbsp. almond flour
- 1 tbsp. Greek full-Fat: yogurt
- 1/8 tsp. baking powder
- ¼ cup swiss cheese crushed

For Filling the Sandwich:

- 3 ounces roast pork
- 2 once deli ham
- 1 slice Swiss cheese
- Chips 3 to 5 pickles, sliced
- ½ tbsp. Dijon mustard

Directions:

1. Preheat your waffle iron.
2. Whisk egg, yogurt, almond flour, and baking powder together.
3. Scatter one-fourth of the Swiss shredded straight onto the hot waffle iron. Cover with half of the mixture of egg, then apply ¼ more Swiss on it. Cover the iron and cook until lightly brown and crunchy for 3-5 minutes.
4. Repeat the same procedure with the ingredients left behind.
5. For the fillings in a sandwich.
6. In a small microwaveable dish, place the pork, Swiss cheese slice, and ham in order. Microwave the cheese for 40 to 50 sec, before it melts.
7. Cover with the mustard on the inner part of one chaffle, then finish with pickles. Reverse the bowl, so the molten Swiss hits the pickles on top of the chaffle. Put the chaffle at the bottom on the roast pork & reverse the sandwich to keep the side of pork below and the side of mustard up.

Nutrition:

- **Calories**: 522
- **Fat**: 33 g
- **Protein**: 46 g
- **Carbohydrates**: 27 g

Preparation Time: 5 minutes

Cooking Time: 7 minutes

Servings: 2

Ingredients:

- 1 egg white
- ¼ cup, shredded (packed) mozzarella cheese
- ¼ cup, shredded (packed) sharp cheddar cheese
- 3/4 tsp. water
- 1 tsp. coconut flour
- ¼ tsp. baking powder
- 1 pinch salt

Directions:

1. Preheat oven to 425°F. Plugin the wall of the Dash Mini Waffle Maker and graze gently until it is hot.
2. Mix all the ingredients in a dish, then mix until combined.
3. At the waffle maker, spoon ½ of the batter out and cover with a lid. Set a 4-minute timer, and do not raise the lid until the cooking period is complete. Preliminary lifting can cause separation of the chaffle keto sandwich recipe and stick to the waffle iron. Before you raise the lid, you have to let it cook the whole 4 minutes.
4. Take the chaffle from the iron, then put it aside. Repeat for the remaining chaffle batter on the same measures above.
5. Position chaffles a few inches apart and cover a baking sheet with parchment paper.
6. Add ¼ to 1/3 cup slow cooker keto roast beef. Before applying to the top of the chaffle, be sure to remove the extra broth/gravy. (Recipes for the slow cooker).
7. Cover with a slice of deli cheese or sliced cheese. Both Swiss and the provolone are fantastic choices.
8. Put on the oven's top rack for 5 minutes to allow the cheese to melt. If you want to bubble the cheese and start browning, set the oven to broil for 1 min. (Swiss cheese does not brown).
9. Enjoy open-faced and dipping with a tiny cup of beef broth.

Nutrition:

- **Calories:** 118
- **Fat:** 8 g
- **Protein:** 9 g
- **Carbohydrates:** 7 g

Preparation Time: 8 minutes

Cooking Time: 7 minutes

Servings: 2

Ingredients:

- 2 chaffles
- Gruyere cheese with thin slices (enough for 3 layers)
- 2 thinly sliced strips ham (or one thicker slice)
- 1-2 tsp. Dijon mustard (or to taste)
- 1 pack keto béchamel sauce

Directions:

1. Make use of the chaffles with the crispy, savory chaffle instructions.
2. The broiler would be preheated on maximum. Put one of the chaffles on a grill rack in a baking dish. Add a layer of gruyere sliced and add a layer of ham sliced. Pour Dijon mustard over the ham. Apply a second layer of grated gruyere over the ham and put the second chaffle over it. Place the béchamel sauce over the top of the sandwich, then place another sliced gruyere layer.
3. Place the sandwich below the broiler before the cheese is melted, bubbly, and light brown. Wait closely to guarantee it's not blackening.
4. Take away from the frying pan. Simply cover with a freshly baked, sunny side up fried egg, served with a touch of salt and pepper if creating it into a Croque Madame. Top it with fresh parsley and enjoy.

Nutrition:

- **Calories:** 360
- **Fat:** 18.4 g
- **Protein:** 7.6 g
- **Carbohydrates:** 8 g

Preparation Time: 5 minutes

Cooking Time: 5 minutes

Servings: 1

Ingredients:

- 1 egg
- 2 slices cheese, thinly sliced
- 1 tsp. natural peanut butter
- 1 tsp. sugar-free raspberry
- Cooking spray

Directions:

1. Crack and whisk the egg in a small bowl or a measuring cup.
2. Lightly grease the waffle maker with cooking spray.
3. Preheat the waffle maker.
4. Once it is heated up, place a slice of cheese on the waffle maker and wait for it to melt.
5. Once melted, pour the egg mixture onto the melted cheese.
6. Once the egg starts cooking, carefully place another slice of cheese on the waffle maker.
7. Close the lid. Cook for 3–4 minutes.
8. Take out the chaffles and place them on a plate.
9. Top the chaffles with whipped cream.
10. Drizzle some natural peanut butter and raspberry preserving on top.

Nutrition:

- **Calories:** 337
- **Carbohydrates:** 3 g
- **Fat:** 27 g
- **Protein:** 9 g

Preparation Time: 3 minutes

Cooking Time: 8 minutes

Servings: 1

Ingredients:

- 1 egg
- ¼ tsp. garlic powder
- ½ cup shred cheddar
- 2 American cheese or ¼ cup shredded cheese
- 1 tbsp. butter

Directions:

1. In a small bowl, mix bacon, garlic powder, and shredded cheddar cheese.
2. After heating the dash waffle maker, add half the mixture of the scramble. Cook for 4 minutes.
3. Add to the dash mini waffle maker the remainder of the scramble mixture and cook for 4 minutes.
4. Steam the stove pan over moderate heat when both chaffles are finished.
5. Attach 1 spoonful of butter and dissolve. Place one chaffle in the pan once the butter has melted. Place your favorite cheese on top of the chaffle and finish with a second chaffle.
6. Cook the chaffle for 1 minute on the first side, turn it over, and cook for another 1–2 minutes on the other side to finish the cheese melting.
7. Cut it from the bread when the cheese melts and eat it!

Nutrition:

- **Calories**: 549
- **Protein**: 27 g
- Fats: 48 g
- **Carbohydrates**: 16 g

Preparation Time: 5 minutes

Cooking Time: 10 minutes

Servings: 1

Ingredients:

- 1 jicama root
- ½ onion, medium, minced
- 2 cloves garlic, pressed
- 1 cup cheese
- 1 egg, whisked
- Salt and pepper

Directions:

1. Peel the jicama root and shred it using a food processor.
2. Place the shredded jicama root in a colander to allow the water to drain. Mix in 2 tsp. of salt as well.
3. Squeeze out the remaining liquid.
4. Microwave the shredded jicama for 5–8 minutes. This step pre-cooks it.
5. Mix all the remaining ingredients together with the jicama.
6. Start preheating the waffle maker.
7. Once preheated, sprinkle a bit of cheese on the waffle maker, allowing it to toast for a few seconds.
8. Place 3 tbsp. of the jicama mixture onto the waffle maker. Sprinkle more cheese on top before closing the lid.
9. Cook for 5 minutes. Flip the chaffle and let it cook for 2 more minutes.
10. Servings your baked jicama by topping it with sour cream, cheese, bacon pieces, and chives.

Nutrition:

- **Calories:** 168
- **Fat:** 11.8 g
- **Protein:** 10 g
- **Carbohydrates:** 16 g

Preparation Time: 5 minutes

Cooking Time: 5 minutes

Servings: 1

Ingredients:

- 1 egg
- ½ cup Monterey jack cheese
- 1 tbsp. almond flour
- 2 tbsp. butter

Directions:

1. Preheat the waffle maker for 5 minutes until it's hot.
2. Combine Monterey jack cheese, almond flour, and the egg in a bowl. Mix well.
3. Take ½ of the batter and pour it into the preheated waffle maker. Allow cooking for 3–4 minutes.
4. Repeat the earlier step for the remaining batter.
5. Melt butter on a small pan. Just like you would with French toast, add the chaffles and let each side cook for 2 minutes. To make them crispier, press down on the chaffles while they cook.
6. Remove the chaffles from the pan. Allow cooling for a few minutes. Servings.

Nutrition:

- **Calories:** 514
- **Fat:** 47 g
- **Protein:** 21 g
- **Carbohydrates:** 19 g

Preparation Time: 5 minutes

Cooking Time: 3-6 minutes

Servings: 1

Ingredients:

- 3 oz. halloumi cheese
- 2 tbsp. pasta sauce

Directions:

1. Make half-inch thick slices of halloumi cheese.
2. With the waffle maker still turned off, place the cheese slices on it.
3. Turn on the waffle maker and let the cheese cook for 3–6 minutes.
4. Remove from the waffle maker and let it cool.
5. Add low-carb pasta or marinara sauce.

Nutrition:

- **Calories:** 333
- **Fat:** 26 g
- **Protein:** 22 g
- **Carbohydrates:** 26 g

97. CHAFFLES BENEDICT

Preparation Time: 15 minutes

Cooking Time: 10 minutes

Servings: 4

Ingredients:

- 12 eggs
- 1 cup cheddar cheese, shredded
- 8 slices bacon
- 3 egg yolks
- 1 tbsp. lemon juice
- 2 pinches kosher salt
- ¼ tsp. Dijon mustard or hot sauce
- ½ cup butter, salted

Directions:

1. Preheat the waffle maker.
2. Pour water in a pan and place over medium-high heat.
3. Take 4 eggs and beat them in a bowl. The remaining eggs are for poaching.
4. Once the waffle maker is heated up, sprinkle 1 tbsp. of cheese and allow it to toast.
5. Take 1 ½ tbsp. of the beaten eggs and place on the toasted cheese.
6. Once the egg starts cooking, add another layer of sprinkled cheese on top.
7. Close the lid. Cook for 2–3 minutes.
8. Remove the cooked chaffle and repeat the steps until you've created 8 chaffles.
9. Fry bacon and set aside for later.
10. Poach the remaining eggs.
11. To make the sauce, combine lemon juice, salt, egg yolks, and Dijon mustard or hot sauce in a bowl.
12. In a separate container, melt the butter in the microwave. Let it cool for a few minutes.
13. Pour the melted butter over the egg yolk mixture.
14. Using an immersion blender, pulse the mixture until it becomes yellow and cloudy. Continue pulsing until the consistency becomes creamy and thick.
15. To Servings, place cooked chaffles on a plate.

16. Place a slice of bacon over each chaffle.

17. Top the bacon with poached egg and drizzle with hollandaise sauce.

Nutrition:

- **Calories**: 601
- **Fat**: 51 g
- **Protein**: 34 g
- **Carbohydrates**: 31 g

Preparation Time: 5 minutes

Cooking Time: 5 minutes

Servings: 1

Ingredients:

- 1 egg, separated
- 1 egg yolk
- ½ cup mozzarella cheese, shredded
- ½ tsp. spiced rum
- 1 tsp. vanilla extract
- ¼ tsp. nutmeg, dried
- A dash cinnamon
- 1 tsp. coconut flour
- 2 tbsp. cream cheese
- 1 tbsp. powdered sweetener
- 2 tsp. rum or rum extract

Directions:

1. Preheat the mini waffle maker.
2. Mix egg yolk in a small bowl until smooth.
3. Add in the sweetener and mix until the powder is completely dissolved.
4. Add the coconut flour, cinnamon, and nutmeg. Mix well.
5. In another bowl, mix rum, egg white, and vanilla. Whisk until well combined.
6. Throw in the yolk mixture with the egg white mixture. You should be able to form a thin batter.
7. Add the mozzarella cheese and combine it with the mixture.
8. Separate the batter into two batches. Put ½ of the batter into the waffle maker and let it cook for 6 minutes until it's solid.
9. Repeat until you've used up the remaining batter.
10. In a separate bowl, mix all the icing ingredients.
11. Top the cooked chaffles with the icing, or you can use this as a dip.

Nutrition:

- **Calories:** 266
- **Fat:** 23 g
- **Protein:** 13 g
- **Carbohydrates:** 11 g

Preparation Time: 10 minutes

Cooking Time: 14 minutes

Servings: 2

Ingredients:

- 1 egg, beaten
- ½ cup finely grated parmesan cheese
- ¼ cup crumbled blue cheese
- 1 tsp. erythritol

Directions:

1. Preheat the waffle iron.
2. Mix all the ingredients in a bowl.
3. Open the iron and add half of the mixture. Close and cook until crispy, 7 minutes.
4. Remove the chaffle onto a plate and make another with the remaining mixture.
5. Cut each chaffle into wedges and Servings afterward.

Nutrition:

- **Calories:** 196
- **Fat:** 13.91 g
- **Protein:** 13.48 g
- **Carbohydrates:** 11 g

Preparation Time: 10 minutes

Cooking Time: 14 minutes

Servings: 2

Ingredients:

- 1 egg, beaten
- ½ cup finely grated cheddar cheese
- ½ cup Greek yogurt for topping
- 8 raspberries and blackberries for topping

Directions:

1. Preheat the waffle iron.
2. Mix the egg and cheddar cheese in a medium bowl.
3. Open the iron and add half of the mixture. Close and cook until crispy, 7 minutes.
4. Remove the chaffle onto a plate and make another with the remaining mixture.
5. Cut each chaffle into wedges and arrange it on a plate.
6. Top each waffle with a tbsp. of yogurt and then two berries.
7. Serve afterward.

Nutrition:

- **Calories:** 207
- **Fat:** 15.29 g
- **Protein:** 12.91 g
- **Carbohydrates:** 16 g

Preparation Time: 10 minutes

Cooking Time: 24 minutes

Servings: 4

Ingredients:

- 1 egg, beaten
- 2 tbsp. swerve brown sugar
- ½ tbsp. butter, melted
- 1 tsp. vanilla extract
- 1 cup finely grated parmesan cheese

Directions:

1. Preheat the waffle iron. Incorporate all the ingredients.
2. Open the iron and pour in a quarter of the mixture. Close and cook until crispy, 6 minutes.
3. Remove the chaffle onto a plate and make 3 more with the remaining ingredients.
4. Cut each chaffle into wedges, plate, allow cooling, and Servings.

Nutrition:

- **Calories:** 136
- **Fat:** 9.45 g
- **Protein:** 8.5 g
- **Carbohydrates:** 6 g

Preparation Time: 10 minutes

Cooking Time: 5 minutes

Servings: 1

Ingredients:

- 1 egg
- 1 oz. cream cheese, softened
- 1 cup cheddar cheese, shredded

For the Toppings:

- 2 tbsp. bacon bits
- ½ tbsp. jalapenos

Directions:

1. Turn on the waffle maker. Preheat for up to 5 minutes.
2. Mix the chaffle ingredients.
3. Pour the batter onto the waffle maker.
4. Cook the batter for 3–4 minutes until it's brown and crispy.
5. Remove the chaffle and repeat steps until all remaining batter has been used up.
6. Sprinkle bacon bits and a few jalapeno slices as toppings.

Nutrition:

- **Calories:** 231
- **Fat:** 18 g
- **Protein:** 13 g
- **Carbohydrates:** 14 g

Preparation Time: 5 minutes

Cooking Time: 5 minutes

Servings: 1

Ingredients:

- 1 egg
- 1/3 cup mozzarella cheese
- ½ cup pork rinds
- Salt

Directions:

1. Preheat the waffle maker.
2. Incorporate a pinch of salt with the cheese, egg, and pork rinds.
3. Pour the mixture onto the preheated waffle maker. Close the lid and wait for 3–5 minutes while it cooks. You'll know it's cooked once it already has a golden-brown color.
4. Carefully remove it from the waffle maker and Servings.

Nutrition:

- **Calories:** 274
- **Fat:** 20 g
- **Protein:** 23 g
- **Carbohydrates:** 16 g

Preparation Time: 5 minutes

Cooking Time: 5 minutes

Servings: 1

Ingredients:

- 1 egg
- ½ cup cheddar cheese, shredded
- 1 tbsp. almond flour
- 1 tbsp. jalapenos
- 1 tbsp. olive oil

Directions:

1. Preheat the waffle maker.
2. While waiting for the waffle maker to heat up, mix jalapeno, egg, cheese, and almond flour in a small mixing bowl.
3. Lightly grease the waffle maker with olive oil.
4. In the center of the waffle maker, carefully pour the chaffle batter. Spread the mixture evenly toward the edges.
5. Close the waffle maker lid and wait for 3-4 minutes for the mixture to cook. For an even crispier texture, wait for another 1–2 minutes.
6. Remove the chaffle. Let it cool before serving.

Nutrition:

- **Calories:** 509
- **Fat:** 45 g
- **Protein:** 23 g
- **Carbohydrates:** 19 g

Preparation Time: 15 minutes

Cooking Time: 32 minutes

Servings: 4

Ingredients:

- 2 eggs
- 1 cup + ¼ cup finely grated cheddar cheese, divided
- 2 chopped fresh scallions
- 2 chicken breasts, cooked and diced
- ¼ cup buffalo sauce
- 3 tbsp. low-carb hummus
- 2 celery stalks, chopped
- ¼ cup crumbled blue cheese for topping

Directions:

1. Preheat the waffle iron.
2. In a medium bowl, mix the eggs, 1 cup of the cheddar cheese, scallions, salt, and black pepper,
3. Open the iron and add a quarter of the mixture. Close and cook until crispy, 7 minutes.
4. Transfer the chaffle to a plate and make 3 more chaffles in the same manner.
5. Prep the oven to 400°F, then prep the baking sheet using parchment paper. Set aside.
6. Cut the chaffles into quarters and arrange them on the baking sheet.
7. Incorporate chicken with buffalo sauce, hummus, and celery.
8. Spoon the chicken mixture onto each quarter of chaffles and top with the remaining cheddar cheese.
9. Put the baking sheet in the oven and bake until the cheese melts, 4 minutes.
10. Take it out from the oven and sprinkle it with the blue cheese.
11. Servings afterward.

Nutrition:

- **Calories**: 552
- **Fat**: 28.37 g
- **Protein**: 59.8 g
- **Carbohydrates**: 26 g

Preparation Time: 20 minutes

Cooking Time: 28 minutes

Servings: 4

Ingredients:

Ingredients:

- 2 eggs, beaten
- 1 cup finely grated cheddar cheese
- ¼ tsp. baking powder
- 2 cups cooked and shredded pork
- 1 tbsp. sugar-free BBQ sauce
- 2 cups shredded coleslaw mix
- 2 tbsp. apple cider vinegar
- ½ tsp. salt
- ¼ cup ranch dressing

Directions:

1. Preheat the waffle iron.
2. In a medium bowl, mix the eggs, cheddar cheese, and baking powder.
3. Open the iron and add a quarter of the mixture. Close and cook until crispy, 7 minutes.
4. Transfer the chaffle to a plate and make 3 more chaffles in the same manner.
5. Meanwhile, in another medium bowl, mix the pulled pork with the BBQ sauce until well combined. Set aside.
6. Also, mix the coleslaw mix, apple cider vinegar, salt, and ranch dressing in another medium bowl.
7. When the chaffles are ready, on two pieces, divide the pork and then top with the ranch coleslaw. Cover with the remaining chaffles and insert mini skewers to secure the sandwiches.
8. Enjoy afterward.

Nutrition:

- **Calories:** 374
- **Fat:** 23.61 g
- **Protein:** 28.05 g
- **Carbohydrates:** 24 g

107. OKONOMIYAKI CHAFFLES

Preparation Time: 20 minutes

Cooking Time: 28 minutes

Servings: 4

Ingredients:

- 2 eggs, beaten
- 1 cup finely grated mozzarella cheese
- ½ tsp. baking powder
- ¼ cup shredded radishes
- 2 tsp. coconut amino
- 2 tbsp. sugar-free ketchup
- 1 tbsp. sugar-free maple syrup
- 2 tsp. Worcestershire sauce
- 1 tbsp. mayonnaise
- 2 tbsp. chopped fresh scallions
- 2 tbsp. bonito flakes
- 1 tsp. dried seaweed powder
- 1 tbsp. pickled ginger

Directions:

For the Chaffles:

1. Preheat the waffle iron.
2. In a medium bowl, mix the eggs, mozzarella cheese, baking powder, and radishes.
3. Open the iron and add a quarter of the mixture. Close and cook until crispy, 7 minutes.
4. Transfer the chaffle to a plate and make a 3 more chaffles in the same manner.

For the Sauce:

1. Combine the coconut amino, ketchup, maple syrup, and Worcestershire sauce in a medium bowl and mix well.

For the Topping:

1. In another mixing bowl, mix the mayonnaise, scallions, bonito flakes, seaweed powder, and ginger

To Servings:

1. Arrange the chaffles on four different plates and swirl the sauce on top. Spread the topping on the chaffles and Servings afterward.

Nutrition:

- **Calories**: 90
- **Fat**: 3.32 g
- **Protein**: 12.09 g
- **Carbohydrates**: 13 g

Preparation Time: 15 minutes

Cooking Time: 28 minutes

Servings: 4

Ingredients:

- 2 eggs, beaten
- 1 cup finely grated swiss cheese
- 2 tsp. caraway seeds
- 1/8 tsp. salt
- ½ tsp. baking powder
- 2 tbsp. sugar-free ketchup
- 3 tbsp. mayonnaise
- 1 tbsp. dill relish
- 1 tsp. hot sauce
- 6 oz. pastrami
- 2 swiss cheese slices
- ¼ cup pickled radishes

Directions:

For the Chaffles:
1. Preheat the waffle iron.
2. In a medium bowl, mix the eggs, Swiss cheese, caraway seeds, salt, and baking powder.
3. Open the iron and add a quarter of the mixture. Close and cook until crispy, 7 minutes.
4. Transfer the chaffle to a plate and make 3 more chaffles in the same manner.

For the Sauce:
1. In another bowl, mix the ketchup, mayonnaise, dill relish, and hot sauce.

To Assemble:
1. Divide on two chaffles; the sauce, the pastrami, Swiss cheese slices, and pickled radishes.
2. Cover with the other chaffles, divide the sandwich into halves, and Servings.

Nutrition:

- **Calories**: 316
- **Fat**: 18 g
- **Protein**: 9 g
- **Carbohydrates**: 10 g

Preparation Time: 15 minutes

Cooking Time: 14 minutes

Servings: 2

Ingredients:

- 2 eggs, beaten
- 1 cup finely grated gruyere cheese
- 2 tbsp. finely grated cheddar cheese
- 1/8 tsp. freshly ground black pepper
- 3 tbsp. minced fresh chives + more for garnishing
- 2 sunshine fried eggs for topping

Directions:

1. Preheat the waffle iron.
2. In a medium bowl, mix the eggs, cheeses, black pepper, and chives.
3. Open the iron and pour in half of the mixture.
4. Close the iron and cook until brown and crispy, 7 minutes.
5. Remove the chaffle onto a plate and set it aside.
6. Make another chaffle using the remaining mixture.
7. Top each chaffle with one fried egg each, garnish with the chives, and Servings.

Nutrition:

- **Calories:** 712
- **Fat:** 41.32 g
- **Protein:** 23.75 g
- **Carbohydrates:** 25 g

Preparation Time: 10 minutes

Cooking Time: 14 minutes

Servings: 2

Ingredients:

- 1 egg, beaten
- ¼ tsp. taco seasoning
- 1/3 cup finely grated cheddar cheese
- 1/3 cup cooked chopped chicken

Directions:

1. Preheat the waffle iron.
2. In a medium bowl, mix the eggs, taco seasoning, and cheddar cheese. Add the chicken and combine well.
3. Open the iron, lightly grease with Cooking spray, and pour in half of the mixture.
4. Close the iron and cook until brown and crispy, 7 minutes.
5. Remove the chaffle onto a plate and set it aside.
6. Make another chaffle using the remaining mixture.
7. Servings afterward.

Nutrition:

- **Calories:** 314
- **Fat:** 20.64 g
- **Protein:** 16.74 g
- **Carbohydrates:** 16 g

Preparation Time: 5 minutes

Cooking Time: 5 minutes

Servings: 2

Ingredients:

- ½ cup canned chicken breast
- ¼ cup cheddar cheese
- 1/8 cup parmesan cheese
- 1 egg
- 1 diced jalapeno (raw or pickled)
- 1/8 tsp. onion powder
- 1/8 tsp. garlic powder
- 1 tsp. cream cheese

Directions:

1. Preheat mini waffle maker.
2. In an average bowl, add all ingredients and stir together till it's completely incorporated.
3. Half this mixture and pour a part of the mixture into a mini waffle maker, and cook for a minimum of five minutes.

Nutrition:

- **Calories:** 224
- **Fat:** 21.8 g
- **Protein:** 18.5 g
- **Carbohydrates:** 16 g

Preparation Time: 10 minutes

Cooking Time: 20 minutes

Servings: 6

Ingredients:

- 2 cups almond flour
- 2 tsp. cinnamon powder
- 1 tbsp. baking soda
- ½ tsp. vanilla extract
- 11 ounces soft tofu, non-GMO, crumbled
- ½ cup butter, melted
- 4 tbsp. stevia
- 1 tbsp. espresso

Directions:

1. In a bowl, mix the flour with baking soda and cinnamon and stir.
2. In your blender, mix tofu with espresso and the other ingredients, pulse well, add to the flour mix and stir until you obtain a batter.
3. Heat up the waffle iron, pour 1/6 of the batter and cook for 6 minutes.
4. Do with the rest of the batter and serve the chaffles cold.

Nutrition:

- **Calories:** 220
- **Fat:** 8 g
- **Protein:** 6 g
- **Carbohydrates:** 6 g

Preparation Time: 10 minutes

Cooking Time: 10 minutes

Servings: 8

Ingredients:

- 1 and ¾ cup almond flour
- 2 tsp. baking powder
- ¼ cup swerve
- ¼ cup Fat-Free Greek yogurt
- ¼ cup coconut butter
- 2 eggs, whisked
- 2 tbsp. cream cheese, soft
- ½ cup cranberries
- 1 tsp. vanilla extract

Directions:

1. Mix flour with the baking powder and the other ingredients and whisk.
2. Preheat the waffle iron, pour 1/8 of the batter and cook for 5 minutes.
3. Repeat with the rest of the batter and serve the chaffles cold.

Nutrition:

- **Calories:** 200
- **Fat:** 6 g
- **Protein:** 7 g
- **Carbohydrates:** 4 g

Preparation Time: 10 minutes

Cooking Time: 10 minutes

Servings: 6

Ingredients:

- 2 eggs, whisked
- 2 tbsp. cream cheese, soft
- 1 cup almond butter
- 1 tsp. almond extract
- ¼ cup almond flour
- 2 tbsp. stevia
- ½ tsp. baking soda

Directions:

1. Mix cream cheese with the almond butter and the other ingredients and whisk.
2. Heat up the waffle iron, pour 1/6 of the batter and cook for 7 minutes.
3. Repeat with the rest of the batter, divide the chaffles between the plates and serve.

Nutrition:

- **Calories:** 140
- **Fat:** 3 g
- **Protein:** 8 g
- **Carbohydrates:** 6 g

Preparation Time: 5 minutes

Cooking Time: 5 minutes

Servings: 4

Ingredients:

- 2 cups coconut flour
- ½ cup cream cheese, soft
- ½ cup fat-free yogurt
- ½ tsp. baking soda
- 1 tsp. baking powder
- 2 tbsp. stevia
- 2 eggs, whisked
- 3 tbsp. coconut oil, melted

Directions:

1. Mix flour with the yogurt and the other ingredients and whisk well.
2. Pour ¼ of the batter in your waffle iron, close, and cook for 5 minutes.
3. Repeat this with the rest of the batter and serve your chaffles right away.

Nutrition:

- **Calories**: 200
- **Fat**: 10 g
- **Protein**: 6 g
- **Carbohydrates**: 7 g

Preparation Time: 10 minutes

Cooking Time: 20 minutes

Servings: 4

Ingredients:

- 2 tbsp. stevia
- 1 and ¼ cup coconut milk
- ¼ cup coconut oil, melted
- ½ tsp. almond extract
- 1 cup almond flour
- ½ cup coconut flour
- 1 and ½ tsp. baking powder
- ¼ tsp. cinnamon powder

For the Syrup:

- 1 and 1/3 cup raspberries
- 4 tbsp. lemon juice
- ½ cup water

Directions:

1. Mix stevia with coconut oil, milk, and the other ingredients except for the syrup and whisk.
2. Pour ¼ of the batter in your waffle iron, cover, and cook for about 5 minutes.
3. Transfer to a plate and repeat with the rest of the batter.
4. Meanwhile, combine the raspberries with lemon juice and the water, whisk heat up over medium heat for 10 minutes.
5. Drizzle the raspberry mix over your chaffles and serve.

Nutrition:

- **Calories**: 230
- **Fat**: 6 g
- **Protein**: 10 g
- **Carbohydrates**: 5 g

Preparation Time: 6 minutes

Cooking Time: 5 minutes

Servings: 4

Ingredients:

- 1 tbsp. coconut oil, melted
- 1 cup almond flour
- 1 egg, whisked
- 3 tbsp. cream cheese, soft
- 1 and ½ cups almond milk
- 3 tbsp. stevia
- 2 tbsp. pumpkin seeds
- 1 tsp. vanilla extract
- 1 tsp. baking soda

Directions:

1. Mix melted coconut oil with the flour and the other ingredients and whisk well.
2. Heat up the waffle iron, pour ¼ of the batter and cook for 5 minutes.
3. Repeat with the rest of the batter and serve the chaffles cold.

Nutrition:

- **Calories:** 220
- **Fat:** 4 g
- **Protein:** 6 g
- **Carbohydrates:** 5 g

Preparation Time: 10 minutes

Cooking Time: 10 minutes

Servings: 6

Ingredients:

- 1 cup coconut flour
- ½ cup cream cheese, soft
- ½ tsp. nutmeg, ground
- 1 cup almond flour
- 3 eggs, whisked
- ¼ cup almond butter, melted

Directions:

1. Mix flour with the cream cheese and the other ingredients and whisk.
2. Heat up the waffle iron, pour 1/6 of the batter and cook for 7 minutes.
3. Repeat with the rest of the batter and serve.

Nutrition:

- **Calories:** 200
- **Fat:** 3 g
- **Protein:** 8 g
- **Carbohydrates:** 6 g

Preparation Time: 10 minutes

Cooking Time: 10 minutes

Servings: 6

Ingredients:

- 1 cup almond flour
- 1 tsp. baking powder
- ½ cup heavy cream
- 3 tbsp. cream cheese, soft
- 1 tsp. baking soda
- 3 tbsp. coconut oil, melted
- 1 cup almond milk
- 3 tbsp. stevia
- ¼ cup lemon juice

Directions:

1. Mix flour with the cream and the other ingredients and whisk well.
2. Heat up the waffle iron, pour 1/6 of the batter and cook for 7 minutes.
3. Repeat with the rest of the batter and serve cold.

Nutrition:

- **Calories**: 346
- **Fat**: 7 g
- **Protein**: 2 g
- **Carbohydrates**: 5 g

Preparation Time: 10 minutes

Cooking Time: 10 minutes

Servings: 8

Ingredients:

- ¼ cup cream cheese, soft
- 2 eggs, whisked
- 1 cup coconut flour
- ½ cup coconut milk
- 3 tbsp. ghee, melted
- ¼ tsp. vanilla extract
- ¼ tsp. peppermint extract

Directions:

1. Mix cream cheese with the eggs and the other ingredients and whisk well.
2. Heat up the waffle iron, pour 1/8 of the batter and cook for 6 minutes.
3. Repeat with the rest of the batter and serve the peppermint chaffles cold.

Nutrition:

- **Calories**: 170
- **Fat**: 2 g
- **Protein**: 4.4 g
- **Carbohydrates**: 1.6 g

Preparation Time: 10 minutes

Cooking Time: 10 minutes

Servings: 6

Ingredients:

- 1/3 cup almond butter, melted
- Juice and zest 1 lime
- 1 cup almond flour
- ½ cup almond milk
- 3 tbsp. cream cheese, soft
- 1 egg, whisked
- 1 tbsp. stevia
- 1 and ½ tbsp. coconut oil

Directions:

1. In a bowl, combine the almond butter with the lime juice, zest, and the other ingredients and whisk well.
2. Heat up the waffle iron, pour 1/6 of the batter inside and cook for 7 minutes.
3. Repeat with the rest of the batter and serve the chaffles cold.

Nutrition:

- **Calories:** 182
- **Fat:** 4 g
- **Protein:** 5.4 g
- **Carbohydrates:** 6 g

Preparation Time: 10 minutes

Cooking Time: 10 minutes

Servings: 6

Ingredients:

- 1 and ¾ cup coconut flour
- Zest from 1 lime, grated
- ¼ cup blackberries
- ¼ cup cranberries
- 2 tsp. baking powder
- ¼ cup swerve
- ¼ cup heavy cream
- ¼ cup cream cheese, warm
- 2 eggs, whisked
- 1 tsp. vanilla extract

Directions:

1. Incorporate flour with the berries, lime zest, and the other ingredients and whisk well.
2. Heat up the waffle iron, pour 1/6 of the batter and cook for 8 minutes.
3. Repeat with the rest of the batter and serve.

Nutrition:

- **Calories:** 200
- **Fat:** 6 g
- **Protein:** 7 g
- **Carbohydrates:** 4 g

Preparation Time: 10 minutes

Cooking Time: 10 minutes

Servings: 6

Ingredients:

- ½ cup almond flour
- ½ cup almond milk
- ½ cup coconut flour
- ½ cup cream cheese, soft
- 2 eggs, whisked
- 1 plum, pitted and chopped
- 1 avocado, peeled, pitted, and chopped
- 1 mango, peeled, pitted, and chopped
- ¼ tsp. cinnamon, ground
- ½ tsp. baking powder

Directions:

1. In your food processor, combine the flour with the milk, cream cheese, and the other ingredients and pulse well.
2. Heat up the waffle iron over medium-high heat, pour 1/6 of the batter and cook for 8 minutes.
3. Repeat with the rest of the batter and serve the chaffles cold.

Nutrition:

- **Calories:** 240
- **Fat:** 4 g
- **Protein:** 6.5 g
- **Carbohydrates:** 8 g

Preparation Time: 10 minutes

Cooking Time: 8 minutes

Servings: 6

Ingredients:

- 1 cup almond flour
- 1 cup coconut cream
- 2 tbsp. chia seeds
- ¼ cup cream cheese, soft
- ¼ tsp. almond extract
- ½ tsp. baking soda
- 1 and ½ tsp. baking powder
- 2 tbsp. swerve
- 2 eggs
- 3 tbsp. coconut oil, melted

Directions:

1. In a bowl, combine the flour with the cream, cream cheese, and the other ingredients and whisk well.
2. Pour 1/6 of the batter in your waffle iron, close, and cook for 6 minutes.
3. Repeat this with the rest of the batter and serve.

Nutrition:

- **Calories:** 200
- **Fat:** 10 g
- **Protein:** 6 g
- **Carbohydrates:** 8 g

Preparation Time: 5 minutes

Cooking Time: 8 minutes

Servings: 6

Ingredients:

- 1 cup almond flour
- 3 tbsp. tomato passata
- 1 cup cream cheese, soft
- 2 eggs, whisked
- 1 tbsp. stevia
- 1 tsp. avocado oil
- ½ cup coconut cream
- 1 tbsp. coconut butter, melted

Directions:

1. In a bowl, combine the flour with the passata and the other ingredients and whisk well.
2. Pour 1/6 of the batter into the heated waffle maker and cook for 8 minutes.
3. Repeat with the rest of the batter and serve.

Nutrition:

- **Calories:** 220
- **Fat:** 4 g
- **Protein:** 4.5 g
- **Carbohydrates:** 6 g

Preparation Time: 5 minutes

Cooking Time: 10 minutes

Servings: 4

Ingredients:

- 1 tbsp. coconut oil, melted
- 1 and ½ cups almond milk
- 1 cup cauliflower rice
- 3 tbsp. stevia
- ½ cup almond flour
- ½ cup cream cheese, soft
- 1 egg, whisked
- 1 tsp. vanilla extract
- 1 tsp. baking soda

Directions:

1. Mix almond milk with the cauliflower rice and the other ingredients and whisk well.
2. Pour ¼ of the batter into the waffle iron, cook for 8 minutes and transfer to a plate.
3. Repeat with the rest of the batter and serve the chaffles warm.

Nutrition:

- **Calories:** 220
- **Fat:** 4 g
- **Protein:** 5.6 g
- **Carbohydrates:** 4 g

Preparation Time: 10 minutes

Cooking Time: 10 minutes

Servings: 4

Ingredients:

- ½ cup mango, peeled and cubed
- 1 cup blueberries
- 1 cup almond flour
- ½ cup cream cheese, soft
- 2 eggs, whisked
- 1 tbsp. heavy cream
- 1 tsp. baking powder
- 3 tbsp. cashew butter

Directions:

1. Mix mango with the berries and the other ingredients and whisk well.
2. Pour ¼ of the batter into the waffle iron, cook for 7 minutes and transfer to a plate.
3. Repeat with the rest of the batter and serve the chaffles warm.

Nutrition:

- **Calories**: 200
- **Fat**: 3 g
- **Protein**: 11 g
- **Carbohydrates**: 9 g

Preparation Time: 10 minutes

Cooking Time: 10 minutes

Servings: 4

Ingredients:

- 1 cup almond flour, GF
- 2 tbsp. ghee, melted
- 1 cup almond milk
- ½ cup cream cheese, soft
- 2 eggs, whisked
- 1 tsp. cinnamon powder
- 1 tsp. nutmeg, ground
- 1 tsp. turmeric powder
- 2 tbsp. heavy cream

Directions:

1. In a bowl, combine the flour with the cream cheese and the other ingredients and whisk well.
2. Pour ¼ of the batter into the waffle iron and cook for 7 minutes.
3. Repeat with the rest of the batter and serve.

Nutrition:

- **Calories:** 220
- **Fat:** 3 g
- **Protein:** 11 g
- **Carbohydrates:** 8 g

Preparation Time: 10 minutes

Cooking Time: 10 minutes

Servings: 4

Ingredients:

- 1 cup coconut milk
- 1 cup almond flour
- 1 cup cashews, soaked for 8 hours in water, and drained
- 2 tbsp. lemon juice
- 2 tbsp. heavy cream
- 1 egg, whisked
- 1 tsp. vanilla extract
- 2 tbsp. cream cheese, soft
- ½ tsp. baking powder

Directions:

1. In your food processor, combine the flour with the cashews and the other ingredients and pulse well.
2. Heat up the waffle iron, pour ¼ of the batter and cook for 7 minutes.
3. Repeat with the rest of the batter and serve the chaffles warm.

Nutrition:

- **Calories**: 200
- **Fat**: 5.6 g
- **Protein**: 5.3 g
- **Carbohydrates**: 4 g

Preparation Time: 10 minutes

Cooking Time: 10 minutes

Servings: 2

Ingredients:

- 1 cup blueberries
- 1 cup coconut flour
- 1 cup coconut cream
- 3 tbsp. cream cheese, soft
- 2 tbsp. stevia
- 1 egg, whisked
- 3 tbsp. almond milk
- 1 tbsp. hemp seeds
- 1 tbsp. chia seeds

Directions:

1. In your blender, combine the berries with the cream, flour, and the other ingredients and mix. Heat up the waffle iron, pour half of the batter and cook for 8 minutes.
2. Repeat with the rest of the batter and serve the chaffles cold.

Nutrition:

- **Calories:** 200
- **Fat:** 2 g
- **Protein:** 3 g
- **Carbohydrates:** 1.6 g

Preparation Time: 10 minutes

Cooking Time: 10 minutes

Servings: 2

Ingredients:

- 1 tsp. cinnamon powder
- 1 cup almond flour
- 1 egg, whisked
- ¼ cup macadamia nuts, chopped
- 1 cup almond milk
- 1 tbsp. cream cheese, soft
- 2 tbsp. coconut flour
- 1 tsp. almond extract
- ½ tbsp. ghee, melted

Directions:

1. In a bowl, combine the flour with the egg, nuts, and the other ingredients and mix.
2. Heat up the waffle iron, pour ½ of the batter and cook for 9 minutes.
3. Repeat with the rest of the batter and serve your chaffles warm.

Nutrition:

- **Calories**: 200
- **Fat**: 5 g
- **Protein**: 4 g
- **Carbohydrates**: 2 g

Preparation Time: 3 minutes

Cooking Time: 7 minutes

Servings: 2

Ingredients:

- ½ cup cheddar cheese, finely shredded
- 1 egg
- 3 drops Pandan extract
- 1 tbsp. almond flour
- 1/3 tsp. garlic powder

Directions:

1. Warm-up your mini waffle maker.
2. Mix the egg, almond flour, garlic powder with cheese in a small bowl.
3. Add Pandan extract to the cheese mixture and mix well.
4. For a crispy crust, add a tsp. of shredded cheese to the waffle maker and cook for 30 seconds.
5. Fill in the mixture into the waffle maker and cook for 5 minutes or until crispy.
6. Repeat with the remaining batter.
7. Serve with fried chicken wings with BBQ sauce and enjoy!

Nutrition:

- **Calories:** 170
- **Fats:** 13 g
- **Protein:** 11 g
- **Carbohydrates:** 9 g

Preparation Time: 5 minutes

Cooking Time: 9 minutes

Servings: 2

Ingredients:

- 2 lbs. cheddar cheese, finely grated
- 2 large eggs
- ½ jalapeno pepper, finely grated
- 2 ounces ham steak
- 1 medium scallion
- 2 tsp. coconut flour

Directions:

1. Shred the cheddar cheese using a fine grater.
2. Deseed the jalapeno and grate using the same grater.
3. Finely chop the scallion and ham.
4. Pour all the ingredients into a medium bowl and mix well.
5. Spray your waffle iron with cooking spray and heat for 3 minutes.
6. Pour ¼ of the batter mixture into the waffle iron.
7. Cook for 3 minutes until crispy around the edges.
8. Remove the waffles from the heat and repeat until all the batter is finished.
9. Once done, allow them to cool to room temperature and enjoy.

Nutrition:

- **Calories:** 120
- **Fat:** 10 g
- **Protein:** 12 g
- **Carbohydrates:** 8 g

134. Hot Ham Chaffles

Preparation Time: 5 minutes

Cooking Time: 4 minutes

Servings: 2

Ingredients:

- ½ cup mozzarella cheese, shredded
- 1 egg
- ¼ cup ham, chopped
- ¼ tsp. salt
- 2 tbsp. mayonnaise
- 1 tsp. Dijon mustard

Directions:

1. Preheat your waffle iron.
2. In the meantime, add the egg to a small mixing bowl and whisk.
3. Add in the ham, cheese, and salt. Mix to combine.
4. Scoop half the mixture using a spoon and pour into the hot waffle iron.
5. Close and cook for 4 minutes.
6. Remove the waffle and place it on a large plate. Repeat the process with the remaining batter.
7. Blend mayo and mustard. Mix together until smooth.
8. Slice the waffles in quarters and use the mayo mixture as the dip.

Nutrition:

- **Calories:** 110
- **Fat:** 12 g
- **Protein:** 12 g
- **Carbohydrates:** 9 g

Preparation Time: 12 minutes

Cooking Time: 10 minutes

Servings: 2

Ingredients:

For the Cheeseburgers:

- 1/3 lb. beef, ground
- ½ tsp. garlic salt
- 3 slices American cheese

For the Chaffles:

- 1 large egg
- ½ cup mozzarella, finely shredded
- Salt and ground pepper to taste

For the Big Mac Sauce:

- 2 tsp. mayonnaise
- 1 tsp. ketchup

To Assemble:

- 2 tbsp. lettuce, shredded
- 4 dill pickles
- 2 tsp. onion, minced

Directions:

Burgers:

1. Heat a pan over medium-high heat.
2. Divide your ground beef into 2 equal balls. Press them to form patties and sprinkle salt and pepper on top. Place balls on the heated griddle and cook for 3 minutes on each side.
3. Place the cheese slices on top of each patty.
4. Proceed to stack them on top of each other and set them aside.

Chaffles:

1. Prep the waffle iron and grease with cooking spray.

2. Stir in the egg, cheese, and salt in a small mixing bowl. Whisk together until well combined.

3. Pour half of the egg mixture into the waffle iron. Cook for 3 minutes.

4. Set aside and repeat the process with the remaining batter.

Big Mac Sauce:

1. Mix together all the ingredients and whisk properly until combined.

To Assemble Burgers:

1. Take your burger patties and place them on one chaffle. Top with shredded lettuce, onions, and pickles.

2. Spread the sauce over the other chaffle and place it on top of the veggies, sauce side down.

3. Enjoy.

Nutrition:

- **Calories**: 850
- **Fat**: 56 g
- **Protein**: 67 g
- **Carbohydrates**: 36 g

Preparation Time: 5 minutes

Cooking Time: 7 minutes

Servings: 2

Ingredients:

- 1 egg
- ½ cup mozzarella cheese, shredded
- A pinch Italian seasoning
- 1 tbsp. sugar-free pizza sauce
- Shredded cheese for topping
- Pepperoni, sliced for topping

Directions:

1. Preheat your waffle maker.
2. Mix the egg and the Italian seasoning together in a small bowl.
3. Add in the shredded cheese and mix.
4. Pour half of the egg mixture into the waffle pan and cook for 5 minutes or until it is golden brown. Once ready, remove the waffle and repeat the process with the remaining mixture.
5. Top the waffle with the pizza sauce, pepperoni, and shredded cheese.
6. Transfer to the microwave and cook on high for 20 seconds.
7. Enjoy your Chaffle pizza!

Nutrition:

- **Calories:** 290
- **Fat:** 22 g
- **Protein:** 24 g
- **Carbohydrates:** 18 g

Preparation Time: 5 minutes

Cooking Time: 10 minutes

Servings: 4

Ingredients:

- 4 eggs
- 1 cup cheddar cheese, shredded
- 8 slices jalapeno, optional
- 1 tsp. red hot sauce
- ¼ tsp. low carb corn extract
- Pinch salt

Directions:

1. Preheat the waffle maker.
2. Beat eggs, then whip.
3. Stir in all the other ingredients and mix thoroughly.
4. Add a pinch of shredded cheese to the hot waffle maker. Cook for 30 seconds.
5. Pour half the egg mixture into the preheated waffle maker.
6. Cook for 5 minutes.
7. Remove, allow to cool, and enjoy.

Nutrition:

- **Calories:** 155
- **Fat:** 12 g
- **Protein:** 10 g
- **Carbohydrates:** 8 g

138. TACO CHAFFLE

Preparation Time: 10 minutes

Cooking Time: 7 minutes

Servings: 2

Ingredients:

Chaffle:

- ½ cup mozzarella, shredded
- 1 egg
- ¼ tsp. Italian seasoning

Taco Meat:

- 1 lb. turkey, ground
- 1 tsp. chili powder
- 1 tsp. cumin, ground
- ½ tsp. garlic powder
- ¼ tsp. onion powder
- ¼ tsp. salt
- ½ tsp. paprika, smoked

Directions:

1. Cook your ground turkey and add all the taco meat seasonings.
2. As the meat cooks, start preparing the chaffles.
3. Preheat your mini waffle maker.
4. Whip the egg in a mixing bowl, add in the cheese and sprinkle with seasoning.
5. Place half of the chaffle mixture into the waffle maker. Cook for 4 minutes.
6. Repeat the process with the second half of the egg mixture.
7. Remove from the waffle maker and add the taco meat on top. To get the perfect taco form you'd better use a taco stand.
8. Top with lettuce, tomatoes, and cheese.
9. Enjoy warm!

Nutrition:

- **Calories:** 120
- **Fat:** 10 g
- **Protein:** 8 g
- **Carbohydrates:** 6 g

Preparation Time: 5 minutes

Cooking Time: 8 minutes

Servings: 2

Ingredients:

Chaffle Bread:

- ½ cup mozzarella cheese, shredded
- 1 egg
- 1 tbsp. green onion, diced
- ½ tsp. Italian seasoning

Sandwich:

- ½ lb. bacon, pre-cooked
- 1 small lettuce
- 1 medium tomato sliced
- 1 tbsp. mayo

Directions:

1. Preheat your mini waffle maker.
2. Whip the egg in a small mixing bowl.
3. Add the seasonings, cheese, and onion. Mix thoroughly until it's well incorporated.
4. Add a tsp. of shredded cheese to the waffle maker and cook for 30 seconds.
5. Place half the batter in the waffle pan and cook for 4 minutes.
6. Once the first chaffle is done, repeat the process with the remaining mixture.
7. Top with mayo, lettuce, bacon, and tomato.
8. Place the second chaffle on top, slice into 2 and enjoy!

Nutrition:

- **Calories**: 240
- **Fat**: 18 g
- **Protein**: 17 g
- **Carbohydrates**: 15 g

Preparation Time: 5 minutes

Cooking Time: 8 minutes

Servings: 2

Ingredients:

- 1 packet tuna, drained
- ½ cup mozzarella cheese
- 1 egg
- A pinch salt

Directions:

1. Preheat the waffle maker.
2. Whip the egg in a small mixing bowl.
3. Add the tuna, cheese, and season with the salt. Mix well.
4. For a crispy crust, add a tsp. of shredded cheese to the waffle maker and cook for 30 seconds.
5. Pour half the mixture into the mini waffle maker and cook for 4 minutes.
6. Remove it and repeat the process with the remaining tuna chaffle mixture.
7. Once ready, remove and enjoy warm.

Nutrition:

- **Calories:** 650
- **Fat:** 39 g
- **Protein:** 63 g
- **Carbohydrates:** 24 g

Preparation Time: 10 minutes

Cooking Time: 17 minutes

Servings: 4

Ingredients:

- 2 eggs
- 1 cup mozzarella cheese, grated
- 4 tbsp. almond flour
- 1 tsp. garlic powder
- 1 tsp. oregano
- ½ tsp. salt

Toppings:

- 4 tbsp. butter, unsalted softened
- ½ tsp. garlic powder
- ½ cup mozzarella cheese, grated

Directions:

1. Preheat your waffle maker.
2. Whisk the eggs in a small bowl.
3. Add the almond flour, mozzarella, oregano, garlic powder, and salt. Mix well.
4. Spoon half the egg mixture into your waffle maker. Cook for 5 minutes and remove.
5. Repeat the process with the remaining batter and cook for 5 minutes.
6. Remove from the waffle maker and cut into 4 strips out of each waffle.
7. Place the waffle sticks on a tray and pre-heat your grill.
8. Add the butter and garlic powder to a small mixing bowl. Mix properly.
9. Using a brush, spread the garlic mixture over the sticks.
10. Sprinkle the shredded mozzarella over the sticks. Place under the grill for 3 minutes or until the cheese starts to melt and bubble.
11. Eat immediately!

Nutrition:

- **Calories**: 109
- **Fat**: 19 g
- **Protein**: 27 g
- **Carbohydrates**: 14 g

Preparation Time: 5 minutes

Cooking Time: 11 minutes

Servings: 2

Ingredients:

- 2 eggs
- 4 tsp. collagen peptides, grass-fed
- 2 tbsp. pork panko
- 3 slices crispy bacon

Directions:

1. Warm-up your mini waffle maker.
2. Combine the eggs, pork panko, and collagen peptides. Mix well. Divide the batter into two small bowls.
3. Once done, evenly distribute ½ of the crispy chopped bacon on the waffle maker.
4. Pour one bowl of the batter over the bacon. Cook for 5 minutes and immediately repeat this step for the second chaffle.
5. Plate your cooked chaffles and sprinkle with extra Panko for an added crunch.
6. Enjoy!

Nutrition:

- **Calories**: 266
- **Fat**: 1 g
- **Protein**: 27 g
- **Carbohydrates**: 15 g

143. Breakfast Chaffle

Preparation Time: 3 minutes

Cooking Time: 4 minutes

Servings: 2

Ingredients:

- 1 large egg
- 2 cup cheese, finely shredded.
- 1,5 tbsp. coconut flour
- 2 tbsp. spring onions
- Salt and pepper to taste

Topping:

- Fried egg
- Scallions, coriander, finely chopped
- BBQ sauce, sugar-free

Directions:

1. Warm-up your mini waffle maker.
2. Incorporate all the ingredients with the exception of topping in a small bowl.
3. Pour the mixture into the waffle maker and cook for 5 minutes or until crispy.
4. Carefully remove.
5. Serve hot topped with the fried egg. Garnish with scallions, coriander, and drizzle with BBQ sauce.
6. Enjoy!

Nutrition:

- **Calories:** 566
- **Fat:** 43 g
- **Protein:** 36 g
- **Carbohydrates:** 24 g

Preparation Time: 6 minutes

Cooking Time: 5 minutes

Servings: 2

Ingredients:

- ½ cup almond milk ricotta, finely shredded
- 1 egg
- 1 cup cauliflower, riced
- ¼ tsp. garlic powder
- ¼ tsp. black pepper, ground
- ½ tsp. Italian seasoning
- ¼ tsp. salt

Directions:

1. Add all the ingredients into a blender. Blend until you have a smooth batter.
2. Evenly spread a spoon of shredded almond milk ricotta into the waffle maker.
3. Pour the cauliflower mixture into the waffle maker.
4. Add another sprinkle of almond milk ricotta on top of the mixture.
5. Cook for 5 minutes or until crispy.
6. Carefully remove and enjoy warm.

Nutrition:

- **Calories:** 270
- **Fat:** 16 g
- **Protein:** 22 g
- **Carbohydrates:** 11 g

Preparation Time: 5 minutes

Cooking Time: 12 minutes

Servings: 2

Ingredients:

- 1 egg
- ½ cup almond milk ricotta, finely shredded.
- 1 tbsp. almond flour
- 2 tbsp. butter

Directions:

1. Mix the egg, almond flour, and ricotta in a small bowl.
2. Separate the chaffle batter into two and cook each for 4 minutes.
3. Cook the butter, then drizzle on top of the chaffles.
4. Put them back in the pan and cook on each side for 2 minutes.
5. Remove from the pan and allow them to sit for 2 minutes.
6. Enjoy while still crispy.

Nutrition:

- **Calories:** 530
- **Fat:** 50 g
- **Protein:** 23 g
- **Carbohydrates:** 18 g

Preparation Time: 5 minutes

Cooking Time: 10 minutes

Servings: 2

Ingredients:

- 2 slices bacon, raw
- 1 egg
- 1 tsp. maple extract, optional
- 1 tsp. all spices

Directions:

1. Put the bacon slices in a blender and turn it on.
2. Once ground up, add in the egg and all spices. Go on blending until liquefied.
3. Heat your waffle maker on the highest setting and spray with non-stick cooking spray.
4. Pour half the omelet into the waffle maker and cook for 5 minutes max.
5. Remove the crispy omelet and repeat the same steps with the rest batter.
6. Enjoy warm.

Nutrition:

- **Calories**: 59
- **Fat**: 4.4 g
- **Protein**: 5 g
- **Carbohydrates**: 6 g

147. Zucchini Chaffles

Preparation Time: 10 minutes

Cooking Time: 7 minutes

Servings: 2

Ingredients:

- ½ cup mozzarella cheese, finely shredded
- 1 egg
- 4 tbsp. parmesan cheese, finely shredded
- 1 cup zucchini, grated
- ¼ tsp. garlic powder
- ¼ tsp. black pepper, ground
- ½ tsp. Italian seasoning
- ¼ tsp. salt

Directions:

1. Season the zucchini with a nip of salt and set it aside for a few minutes. Squeeze out the excess water.
2. Warm-up your mini waffle maker.
3. Mix all the ingredients in a small bowl.
4. For a crispy crust, add a tsp. of shredded cheese to the waffle maker and cook for 30 seconds.
5. Ladle the batter into the waffle maker, then cook for 5 minutes or until crispy.
6. Carefully remove.
7. Enjoy!

Nutrition:

- **Calories:** 190
- **Fat:** 13 g
- **Protein:** 16 g
- **Carbohydrates:** 12 g

Preparation Time: 5 minutes

Cooking Time: 7 minutes

Servings: 2

Ingredients:

- ½ avocado
- 1 egg
- ½ cup cheddar cheese, finely shredded
- 1 tbsp. almond flour
- 1 tsp. lemon juice, fresh
- Salt, ground pepper to taste
- Parmesan cheese, finely shredded for garnishing

Directions:

1. Warm-up your mini waffle maker.
2. Mix the egg, almond flour with cheese in a small bowl.
3. For a crispy crust, add a tsp. of shredded cheese to the waffle maker and cook for 30 seconds.
4. Ladle the batter, then cook for 5 minutes or until crispy.
5. Repeat with the remaining batter.
6. Mash avocado with a fork until well combined and add lemon juice, salt, pepper
7. Top each chaffle with an avocado mixture. Sprinkle with parmesan and enjoy!

Nutrition:

- **Calories:** 250
- **Fat:** 23 g
- **Protein:** 14 g
- **Carbohydrates:** 11 g

Preparation Time: 3 minutes

Cooking Time: 7 minutes

Servings: 2

Ingredients:

- ½ cup cheddar cheese, finely shredded
- 1 egg
- 1/3 cup broccoli, fresh chopped
- 1 tbsp. almond flour
- 1/3 tsp. garlic powder

Directions:

1. Warm-up your mini waffle maker.
2. Mix the egg, almond flour, garlic powder with cheese in a small bowl.
3. Add half broccoli to the cheese mixture.
4. For a crispy crust, add a tsp. of shredded cheese to the waffle maker and cook for 30 seconds.
5. Ladle the batter into the waffle maker, then cook for 5 minutes or until crispy.
6. Repeat with the remaining batter. Serve with a fried slice of bacon and enjoy!

Nutrition:

- **Calories**: 180
- **Fat**: 13 g
- **Protein**: 11 g
- **Carbohydrates**: 9 g

Preparation Time: 5 minutes

Cooking Time: 15 minutes

Servings: 4

Ingredients:

- 2 oz. chicken breasts, cooked, shredded
- ½ cup mozzarella cheese, finely shredded
- 2 eggs
- 6 tbsp. parmesan cheese, finely shredded
- 1 cup zucchini, grated
- ½ cup almond flour
- 1 tsp baking powder
- ¼ tsp. garlic powder
- ¼ tsp. black pepper, ground
- ½ tsp. Italian seasoning
- ¼ tsp. salt

Directions:

1. Season the zucchini with a nip of salt and set it aside for a few minutes. Squeeze out the excess water.
2. Warm-up your mini waffle maker.
3. Mix chicken, almond flour, baking powder, cheeses, garlic powder, salt, pepper, and seasonings in a bowl.
4. Use another small bow for beating eggs. Add them to squeezed zucchini, mix well.
5. Combine the chicken and egg mixture, and mix.
6. For a crispy crust, add a tsp. of shredded cheese to the waffle maker and cook for 30 seconds.
7. Then, pour the mixture into the waffle maker and cook for 5 minutes or until crispy.
8. Carefully remove. Repeat with the remaining batter the same steps.
9. Enjoy!

Nutrition:

- **Calories:** 135
- **Fat:** 10 g
- **Protein:** 11 g
- **Carbohydrates:** 9 g

Preparation Time: 10 minutes

Cooking Time: 27 minutes

Servings: 6

Ingredients:

- 1 lb. crab meat
- 1/3 cup Panko breadcrumbs
- 1 egg
- 2 tbsp. fat Greek yogurt
- 1 tsp. Dijon mustard
- 2 tbsp. parsley and chives, fresh
- 1 tsp. Italian seasoning
- 1 lemon, juiced
- salt, pepper to taste

Directions:

1. Preheat the waffle maker
2. Incorporate all the ingredients, except crab meat.
3. Add the meat. Mix well.
4. Form the mixture into round patties.
5. Cook 1 patty for 3 minutes.
6. Remove it and repeat the process with the remaining crab chaffle mixture.
7. Once ready, remove and enjoy warm.

Nutrition:

- **Calories:** 99
- **Fat:** 8 g
- **Protein:** 16 g
- **Carbohydrates:** 12 g

Chapter 8.

EXPERT CHAFFLE RECIPES

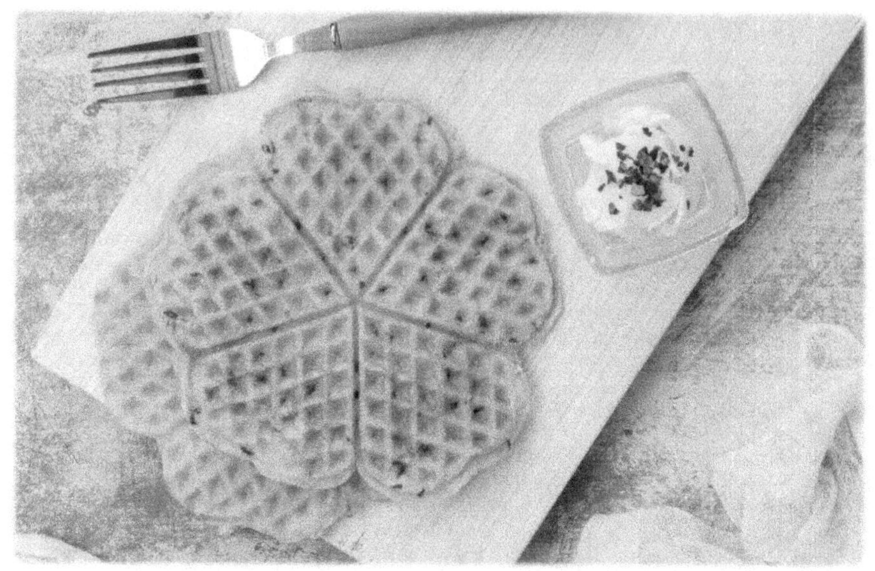

152. HAM, CHEESE & TOMATO CHAFFLE SANDWICH

Preparation Time: 5 minutes

Cooking Time: 10 minutes

Servings: 2

Ingredients:

- 1 tsp. olive oil
- 2 slices ham
- 4 basic chaffles
- 1 tbsp. mayonnaise
- 2 slices Provolone cheese
- 1 tomato, sliced

Directions:

1. Pour in olive oil into a pan at medium heat.

2. Cook the ham for 1 minute per side.

3. Spread the chaffles with mayonnaise.

4. Top with ham, cheese, and tomatoes.

5. Top with another chaffle to make a sandwich.

Nutrition:

- **Calories**: 198
- **Fat**: 14.7 g
- **Protein**: 12.2 g
- **Carbohydrates**: 11 g

Preparation Time: 5 minutes

Cooking Time: 15 minutes

Servings: 2

Ingredients:

- ¼ cup sausage, cooked
- 3 tbsp. chicken broth
- 2 tsp. cream cheese
- 2 tbsp. heavy whipping cream
- ¼ tsp. garlic powder
- Pepper to taste
- 2 basic chaffles

Directions:

1. Add the sausage, broth, cream cheese, cream, garlic powder, and pepper to a pan over medium heat.
2. Allow to boil, then lower the heat.
3. Simmer for 10 minutes until thickened.
4. Pour the gravy on top of the basic chaffles
5. Serve.

Nutrition:

- **Calories**: 212
- **Fat**: 17 g
- **Protein**: 11 g
- **Carbohydrates**: 9 g

Preparation Time: 5 minutes

Cooking Time: 8 minutes

Servings: 2

Ingredients:

- 1 egg, beaten
- ½ cup cheddar cheese, shredded
- ½ tsp. barbecue sauce
- ¼ tsp. baking powder

Directions:

1. Plug in your waffle maker to preheat.
2. Mix all the ingredients in a bowl.
3. Pour half of the mixture into your waffle maker.
4. Cover and cook for 4 minutes.
5. Repeat the same steps for the next barbecue chaffle.

Nutrition:

- **Calories:** 295
- **Fat:** 23 g
- **Protein:** 20 g
- **Carbohydrates:** 14 g

Preparation Time: 5 minutes

Cooking Time: 8 minutes

Servings: 2

Ingredients:

- 1 egg
- ¼ cup chicken cubes, cooked
- 1 slice bacon, cooked and chopped
- ¼ cup cheddar cheese, shredded
- 1 tsp. ranch dressing powder

Directions:

1. Preheat your waffle maker.
2. In a bowl, mix all the ingredients.
3. Pour in half of the batter into your waffle maker.
4. Cover and cook for 4 minutes.
5. Make the second chaffle using the same steps.

Nutrition:

- **Calories:** 200
- **Fat:** 14 g
- **Protein:** 16 g
- **Carbohydrates:** 12 g

Preparation Time: 15 minutes

Cooking Time: 15 minutes

Servings: 2

Ingredients:

- 1 lb. ground beef
- 1 onion, minced
- 1 tsp. parsley, chopped
- 1 egg, beaten
- Salt and pepper to taste
- 1 tbsp. olive oil
- 4 basic chaffles
- 2 lettuce leaves
- 2 cheese slices
- 1 tbsp. dill pickles
- Ketchup
- Mayonnaise

Directions:

1. Incorporate ground beef, onion, parsley, egg, salt and pepper.
2. Mix well.
3. Form 2 thick patties.
4. Add olive oil to the pan.
5. Place the pan over medium heat.
6. Cook the patty for 3 to 5 minutes per side or until fully cooked.
7. Place the patty on top of each chaffle.
8. Top with lettuce, cheese, and pickles.
9. Squirt ketchup and mayo over the patty and veggies.
10. Top with another chaffle.

Nutrition:

- **Calories:** 325
- **Fat:** 16.3 g
- **Protein:** 39.6 g
- **Carbohydrates:** 26 g

Preparation Time: 10 minutes

Cooking Time: 15 minutes

Servings: 2

Ingredients:

- 1 tsp. olive oil
- 2 cups ground beef
- Garlic salt to taste
- 1 red bell pepper, sliced into strips
- 1 green bell pepper, sliced into strips
- 1 onion, minced
- 1 bay leaf
- 2 garlic chaffles
- Butter

Directions:

1. Put your pan over medium heat.
2. Add the olive oil and cook ground beef until brown.
3. Season with garlic salt and add a bay leaf.
4. Drain the fat, transfer it to a plate and set it aside.
5. Discard the bay leaf.
6. In the same pan, cook the onion and bell peppers for 2 minutes.
7. Put the beef back to the pan.
8. Heat for 1 minute.
9. Spread butter on top of the chaffle.
10. Add the ground beef and veggies.
11. Roll or fold the chaffle.

Nutrition:

- **Calories:** 220
- **Fat:** 17.8 g
- **Protein:** 27.1 g
- **Carbohydrates:** 14 g

Preparation Time: 5 minutes

Cooking Time: 5 minutes

Servings: 2

Ingredients:

- 2 basic chaffles
- 2 tbsp. sugar-free marinara sauce
- 2 tbsp. mozzarella, shredded
- 1 tbsp. olives, sliced
- 1 tomato sliced
- 1 tbsp. keto-friendly pesto sauce
- Basil leaves

Directions:

1. Spread marinara sauce on each chaffle.
2. Spoon pesto and spread on top of the marinara sauce.
3. Top with the tomato, olives, and mozzarella.
4. Bake in the oven for 3 minutes or until the cheese has melted.
5. Garnish with basil.
6. Serve and enjoy.

Nutrition:

- **Calories:** 182
- **Fat:** 11 g
- **Protein:** 16.8 g
- **Carbohydrates:** 15 g

Preparation Time: 15 minutes

Cooking Time: 14 minutes

Servings: 2

Ingredients:

- 1 egg, beaten
- 1 cup finely grated cheddar cheese
- 2 hot dog sausages, cooked
- Mustard dressing for topping
- 8 pickle slices

Directions:

1. Preheat the waffle iron.
2. Whisk egg and cheddar cheese.
3. Open the iron and add half of the mixture. Close and cook until crispy, 7 minutes.
4. Transfer the chaffle to a plate and make a second chaffle in the same manner.
5. To serve, top each chaffle with a sausage, swirl the mustard dressing on top, and then divide the pickle slices on top.
6. Enjoy!

Nutrition:

- **Calories:** 231
- **Fat:** 18.29 g
- **Protein:** 13.39 g
- **Carbohydrates:** 11 g

Preparation Time: 15 minutes

Cooking Time: 32 minutes

Servings: 4

Ingredients:

- 2 eggs
- 1 cup + ¼ cup finely grated cheddar cheese, divided
- 2 chopped fresh scallions
- 2 chicken breasts, cooked and diced
- ¼ cup buffalo sauce
- 3 tbsp. low-carb hummus
- 2 celery stalks, chopped
- ¼ cup crumbled blue cheese for topping

Directions:

1. Preheat the waffle iron.
2. In a medium bowl, mix the eggs, 1 cup of the cheddar cheese, scallions, salt, and black pepper,
3. Open the iron and add a quarter of the mixture. Close and cook until crispy, 7 minutes.
4. Transfer the chaffle to a plate and make 3 more chaffles in the same manner.
5. Prep the oven to 400°F, then prep the baking sheet using parchment paper. Set aside.
6. Cut the chaffles into quarters and arrange them on the baking sheet.
7. Incorporate chicken with buffalo sauce, hummus, and celery.
8. Spoon the chicken mixture onto each quarter of chaffles and top with the remaining cheddar cheese.
9. Place the baking sheet in the oven and bake until the cheese melts, 4 minutes.
10. Pull it out from the oven and top with the blue cheese.
11. Serve afterward.

Nutrition:

- **Calories:** 552
- **Fat:** 28.37 g
- **Protein:** 59.8 g
- **Carbohydrates:** 26 g

Preparation Time: 20 minutes

Cooking Time: 28 minutes

Servings: 4

Ingredients:

- 2 eggs, beaten
- 1 cup finely grated cheddar cheese
- ¼ tsp. baking powder
- 2 cups cooked and shredded pork
- 1 tbsp. sugar-free BBQ sauce
- 2 cups shredded coleslaw mix
- 2 tbsp. apple cider vinegar
- ½ tsp. salt
- ¼ cup ranch dressing

Directions:

1. Preheat the waffle iron.
2. In a medium bowl, mix the eggs, cheddar cheese, and baking powder.
3. Open the iron and add a quarter of the mixture. Close and cook until crispy, 7 minutes.
4. Transfer the chaffle to a plate and make 3 more chaffles in the same manner.
5. Meanwhile, in another medium bowl, mix the pulled pork with the BBQ sauce until well combined. Set aside.
6. Also, mix the coleslaw mix, apple cider vinegar, salt, and ranch dressing in another medium bowl.
7. When the chaffles are ready, on two pieces, divide the pork and then top with the ranch coleslaw. Cover with the remaining chaffles and insert mini skewers to secure the sandwiches.
8. Enjoy.

Nutrition:

- **Calories:** 374
- **Fat:** 23.61 g
- **Protein:** 28.05 g
- **Carbohydrates:** 19 g

Preparation Time: 15 minutes

Cooking Time: 28 minutes

Servings: 4

Ingredients:

For the Chaffles:

- 2 eggs, beaten
- 1 cup finely grated Swiss cheese
- 2 tsp. caraway seeds
- 1/8 tsp. salt
- ½ tsp. baking powder

For the Sauce:

- 2 tbsp. sugar-free ketchup
- 3 tbsp. mayonnaise
- 1 tbsp. dill relish
- 1 tsp. hot sauce

For the Filling:

- 6 oz. pastrami
- 2 Swiss cheese slices
- ¼ cup pickled radishes

Directions:

For the Chaffles:

1. Preheat the waffle iron.
2. In a medium bowl, mix the eggs, Swiss cheese, caraway seeds, salt, and baking powder.
3. Open the iron and add a quarter of the mixture. Close and cook until crispy, 7 minutes.
4. Transfer the chaffle to a plate and make 3 more chaffles in the same manner.

For the Sauce:

1. In another bowl, mix the ketchup, mayonnaise, dill relish, and hot sauce.

To Assemble:

1. Divide on two chaffles; the sauce, the pastrami, Swiss cheese slices, and pickled radishes.

2. Cover with the other chaffles, divide the sandwich into halves, and serve.

Nutrition:

- **Calories**: 316
- **Fat**: 21.78 g
- **Protein**: 23.56 g
- **Carbohydrates**: 19 g

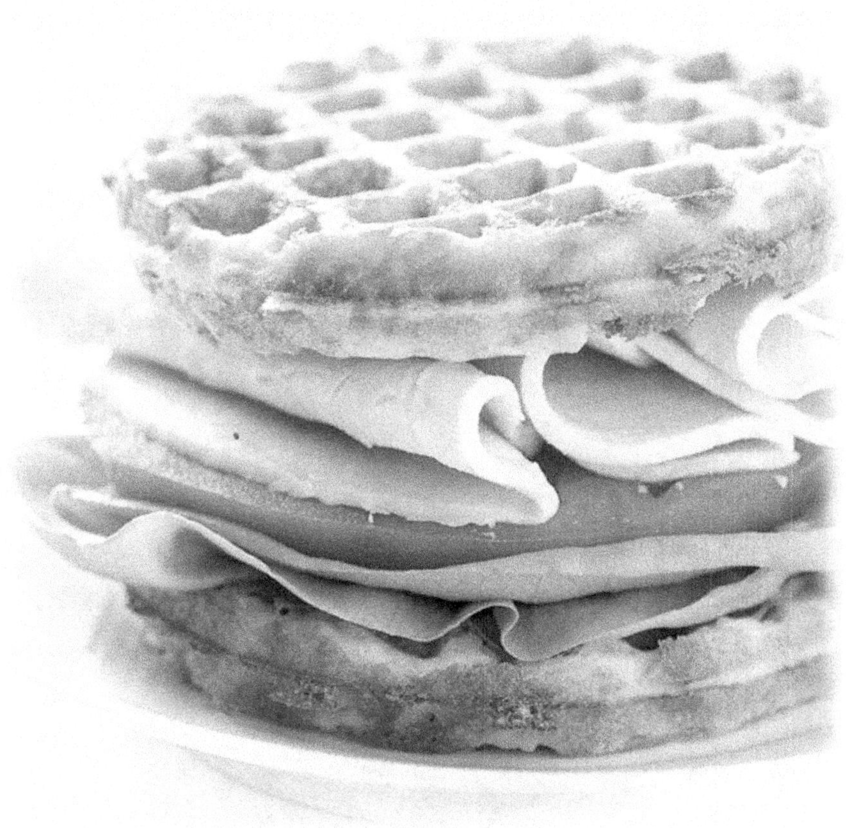

Preparation Time: 15 minutes

Cooking Time: 28 minutes

Servings: 4

Ingredients:

- 1 cup finely shredded parsnips, steamed
- 8 oz. ham, diced
- 2 eggs, beaten
- 1 ½ cups finely grated cheddar cheese
- ½ tsp. garlic powder
- 2 tbsp. chopped fresh parsley leaves
- ¼ tsp. smoked paprika
- ½ tsp. dried thyme

Directions:

1. Prep the waffle iron.
2. Incorporate all the ingredients.
3. Open the iron, lightly grease with cooking spray, and pour in a quarter of the mixture.
4. Close the iron and cook until crispy, 7 minutes.
5. Remove the chaffle onto a plate and set it aside.
6. Make three more chaffles using the remaining mixture.
7. Serve.

Nutrition:

- **Calories:** 506
- **Fat:** 24.05 g
- **Protein:** 42.74 g
- **Carbohydrates:** 36 g

Preparation Time: 15 minutes

Cooking Time: 14 minutes

Servings: 2

Ingredients:

- 2 eggs, beaten
- 1 cup finely grated Gruyere cheese
- 2 tbsp. finely grated cheddar cheese
- 1/8 tsp. freshly ground black pepper
- 3 tbsp. minced fresh chives + more for garnishing
- 2 sunshine fried eggs for topping

Directions:

1. Preheat the waffle iron.
2. In a medium bowl, mix the eggs, cheeses, black pepper, and chives.
3. Open the iron and pour in half of the mixture.
4. Close the iron and cook until brown and crispy, 7 minutes.
5. Remove the chaffle onto a plate and set it aside.
6. Make another chaffle using the remaining mixture.
7. Top each chaffle with one fried egg each, garnish with the chives and serve.

Nutrition:

- **Calories:** 712
- **Fat:** 41.32 g
- **Protein:** 23.75 g
- **Carbohydrates:** 22 g

Preparation Time: 5 minutes

Cooking Time: 8 minutes

Servings: 2

Ingredients:

- 1 egg, beaten
- 1 cup cheddar cheese, shredded
- ¼ cup Parmesan cheese, grated
- 1 lb. Italian sausage, crumbled
- 2 tsp. baking powder
- 1 cup almond flour

Directions:

1. Preheat your waffle maker.
2. Mix all the ingredients in a bowl.
3. Fill in half of the batter into the waffle maker.
4. Cover and cook for 4 minutes.
5. Transfer to a plate.
6. Let cool to make it crispy.
7. Do the same steps to make the next chaffle.

Nutrition:

- **Calories:** 332
- **Fat:** 27.1 g
- **Protein:** 19.6 g
- **Carbohydrates:** 19 g

Preparation Time: 10 minutes

Cooking Time: 15 minutes

Servings: 2

Ingredients:

- Cooking spray
- 4 slices bacon
- 1 tbsp. mayonnaise
- 4 basic chaffles
- 2 lettuce leaves
- 2 tomato slices

Directions:

1. Coat your pan with foil and place it over medium heat.
2. Cook the bacon until golden and crispy.
3. Spread mayo on top of the chaffle.
4. Top with lettuce, bacon, and tomato.
5. Top with another chaffle.

Nutrition:

- **Calories:** 238
- **Fat:** 18.4 g
- **Protein:** 14.3 g
- **Carbohydrates:** 13 g

Preparation Time: 15 minutes

Cooking Time: 15 minutes

Servings: 2

Ingredients:

- 1 tsp. olive oil
- 1 lb. ground beef
- Salt and pepper to taste
- 1 tsp. onion powder
- 1 tsp. garlic powder
- 3 tbsp. tomato paste
- 1 tbsp. chili powder
- 1 tsp. mustard powder
- ½ tsp. paprika
- ½ cup beef broth
- 1 tsp. coconut amino
- 1 tsp. sweetener
- 4 cornbread chaffles

Directions:

1. Drizzle the olive oil into a pan at medium-high heat.
2. Add the ground beef.
3. Season with salt, pepper, and spices.
4. Cook for 5 minutes, stirring occasionally.
5. Stir in the beef broth, coconut aminos, and sweetener.
6. Reduce heat and simmer for 10 minutes.
7. Top the cornbread chaffle with the ground beef mixture.
8. Top with another chaffle.

Nutrition:

- **Calories:** 334
- **Fat:** 12.1 g
- **Protein:** 48.2 g
- **Carbohydrates:** 19 g

168. BACON CHAFFLE

Preparation Time: 5 minutes

Cooking Time: 8 minutes

Servings: 2

Ingredients:

- 1 egg
- ½ cup cheddar cheese, shredded
- 1 tsp. baking powder
- 2 tbsp. almond flour
- 3 tbsp. bacon bits, cooked

Directions:

1. Turn your waffle maker on.
2. Beat the egg in a bowl.
3. Stir in the cheese, baking powder, almond flour, and bacon bits.
4. Fill in half of the batter into the waffle maker.
5. Close the device.
6. Cook for 4 minutes.
7. Open and transfer waffle on a plate. Let cool for 2 minutes.
8. Repeat the same procedure with the remaining batter.

Nutrition:

- **Calories:** 147
- **Fat:** 11.5 g
- **Protein:** 9.8 g
- **Carbohydrates:** 6 g

169. Pizza Flavored Chaffle

Preparation Time: 10 minutes

Cooking Time: 12 minutes

Servings: 3

Ingredients:

- 1 egg, beaten
- ½ cup cheddar cheese, shredded
- 2 tbsp. pepperoni, chopped
- 1 tbsp. keto marinara sauce
- 4 tbsp. almond flour
- 1 tsp. baking powder
- ½ tsp. dried Italian seasoning
- Parmesan cheese, grated

Directions:

1. Preheat your waffle maker.
2. In a bowl, mix the egg, cheddar cheese, pepperoni, marinara sauce, almond flour, baking powder, and Italian seasoning.
3. Add the mixture to the waffle maker.
4. Close the device and cook for 4 minutes.
5. Open it and transfer the chaffle to a plate.
6. Let cool for 2 minutes.
7. Repeat the steps with the remaining batter.
8. Top with the grated Parmesan and serve.

Nutrition:

- **Calories:** 179
- **Fat:** 14.3 g
- **Protein:** 11.1 g
- **Carbohydrates:** 13 g

Preparation Time: 5 minutes

Cooking Time: 8 minutes

Servings: 2

Ingredients:

- 1 egg
- ½ cup Swiss cheese
- 2 tbsp. cooked crumbled bacon

Directions:

1. Preheat your waffle maker.
2. Beat the egg in a bowl.
3. Stir in the cheese and bacon.
4. Pour half of the mixture into the device.
5. Close and cook for 4 minutes.
6. Cook the second chaffle using the same steps.

Nutrition:

- **Calories:** 237
- **Fat:** 17.6 g
- **Protein:** 17.1 g
- **Carbohydrates:** 11 g

Preparation Time: 5 minutes

Cooking Time: 8 minutes

Servings: 2

Ingredients:

- 1 egg
- ½ cup cheddar cheese, shredded
- 1 tbsp. black olives, chopped
- 1 tbsp. bacon bits

Directions:

1. Plug in your waffle maker.
2. In a bowl, beat the egg and stir in the cheese.
3. Add the black olives and bacon bits.
4. Mix well.
5. Add half of the mixture into the waffle maker.
6. Cover and cook for 4 minutes.
7. Open and transfer to a plate.
8. Let cool for 2 minutes.
9. Cook the other chaffle using the remaining batter.

Nutrition:

- **Calories:** 202
- **Fat:** 16 g
- **Protein:** 13.4 g
- **Carbohydrates:** 12 g

Preparation Time: 5 minutes

Cooking Time: 20 minutes

Servings: 2

Ingredients:

- Chicken: 3–4 pieces
- Lemon juice: ½ tbsp.
- Garlic: 1 clove
- Kewpie mayo: 2 tbsp.
- Egg: 1
- Mozzarella cheese: ½ cup
- Salt: As per your taste

Directions:

1. In a pot, cook the chicken by adding one cup of water to it with salt and bring to boil
2. Seal the lid of the pot, then cook for 15–20 minutes
3. When done, remove from stove and shred the chicken pieces leaving the bones behind; discard the bones
4. Grate garlic finely into pieces
5. Beat the egg in the mixing bowl, add garlic, lemon juice, Kewpie mayo, and 1/8 cup of cheese
6. Preheat the waffle maker if needed and grease it
7. Ladle the mixture to the waffle maker and cook for 4–5 minutes or until it is done
8. Remove the chaffles from the pan and preheat the oven
9. In the meanwhile, set the chaffles on a baking tray and spread the chicken on them
10. After that, sprinkle the remaining cheese on the chaffles
11. Put the tray in the oven and heat till the cheese melts
12. Serve hot
13. Make as many chaffles as you like

Nutrition:

- **Calories**: 255
- **Fat**: 21 g
- **Protein**: 18 g
- **Carbohydrates**: 16 g

Preparation Time: 5 minutes

Cooking Time: 10 minutes

Servings: 2

Ingredients:

- 1 cup chicken
- 2 eggs
- 1 cup and 4 tbsp. Mozzarella cheese
- 6 tbsp. tomato sauce
- ½ tsp. basil
- ½ tbsp. garlic
- 1 tsp. butter

Directions:

1. In a pan, add butter and include small pieces of chicken in it.
2. Stir for two minutes, and then add garlic and basil.
3. Set aside the cooked chicken.
4. Preheat the mini waffle maker if needed.
5. Mix cooked chicken, eggs, and 1 cup mozzarella cheese properly.
6. Spread it to the mini waffle maker thoroughly.
7. Cook for 4 minutes or till it turns crispy, and then remove it from the waffle maker.
8. Make as many mini chaffles as you can.
9. Now in a baking tray, line these mini chaffles and top with the tomato sauce and grated mozzarella cheese.
10. Put the tray in the oven at 400°F until the cheese melts.
11. Serve hot.

Nutrition:

- **Calories:** 244
- **Fat:** 11 g
- **Protein:** 13 g
- **Carbohydrates:** 9 g

Preparation Time: 15 minutes

Cooking Time: 17 minutes

Servings: 2

Ingredients:

For Chaffle:

- Egg: 2
- Mozzarella Cheese: 1 cup (shredded)
- Butter: 1 tbsp.
- Almond flour: 2 tbsp.
- Turmeric: ¼ tsp.
- Baking powder: ¼ tsp.
- Xanthan gum: a pinch
- Onion powder: a pinch
- Garlic powder: a pinch
- Salt: a pinch

For Chicken Jamaican Jerk:

- Organic ground chicken: 1 pound
- Dried thyme: 1 tsp.
- Garlic: 1 tsp. (granulated)
- Butter: 2 tbsp.
- Dried parsley: 2 tsp.
- Black pepper: 1/8 tsp.
- Salt: 1 tsp.
- Chicken broth: ½ cup
- Jerk seasoning: 2 tbsp.
- Onion: ½ medium chopped

Directions:

1. In a pan, melt butter and sauté onion.
2. Add all the remaining ingredients of Jamaican chicken jerk and sauté.

3. Now add chicken and chicken broth and stir.

4. Cook on medium-low heat for 10 minutes.

5. Then cook on high heat and dry all the liquid.

6. For chaffles, preheat a mini waffle maker if needed and grease i.t

7. In a mixing bowl, beat all the chaffle ingredients.

8. Pour the mixture to the lower plate of the waffle maker and spread it evenly to cover the plate properly, and close the lid.

9. Cook for at least 4 minutes to get the desired crunch.

10. Remove the chaffle from the heat and keep it aside for around one minute.

11. Make as many chaffles as your mixture and waffle maker allow.

12. Add the chicken in between a chaffle and fold, and enjoy.

Nutrition:

- **Calories**: 262
- **Fat**: 26 g
- **Protein**: 19.4 g
- **Carbohydrates**: 12 g

Preparation Time: 5 minutes

Cooking Time: 10 minutes

Servings: 2

Ingredients:

For Chaffle:

- Chicken: 1/3 cup boiled and shredded
- Cabbage: 1/3 cup
- Broccoli: 1/3 cup
- Zucchini: 1/3 cup
- Egg: 2
- Mozzarella Cheese: 1 cup (shredded)
- Butter: 1 tbsp.
- Almond flour: 2 tbsp.
- Baking powder: ¼ tsp.
- Onion powder: a pinch
- Garlic powder: a pinch
- Salt: a pinch

Directions:

1. Using a deep saucepan, boil cabbage, broccoli, and zucchini for five minutes or till it tenders, strain, and blend.
2. Incorporate all the remaining ingredients well together.
3. Fill in a thin layer on a preheated waffle iron.
4. Stir in a layer of the blended vegetables on the mixture.
5. Mix in more mixture over the top.
6. Allow cooking the chaffle for around 5 minutes.
7. Serve.

Nutrition:

- **Calories**: 312
- **Fat**: 18 g
- **Protein**: 15 g
- **Carbohydrates**: 13 g

176. Chicken Chaffle

Preparation Time: 5 minutes

Cooking Time: 11 minutes

Servings: 2

Ingredients:

- 2 eggs
- 1 cup Cheddar cheese
- 4 tbsp. or to your taste Buffalo sauce
- ¼ cup softened cream cheese
- 1 cup chicken
- 1 tsp. butter

Directions:

1. Heat the butter in the pan and add shredded chicken to it.
2. Now remove from heat and add buffalo sauce as per your taste.
3. In a bowl, add cooked chicken, cheddar cheese, softened cream cheese, and eggs.
4. Mix all the ingredients well.
5. Preheat the waffle maker and grease it.
6. Now sprinkle a little cheddar cheese at the lower plate of the waffle maker.
7. Spread your prepared batter evenly on the waffle maker.
8. Now add a bit of cheese on the top as well and close the lid.
9. Heat the chaffle for over 4 minutes or until it turns crispy.
10. Make as many chaffles as your mixture and waffle maker allow.
11. Serve hot with extra buffalo sauce.

Nutrition:

- **Calories**: 292
- **Fat**: 11 g
- **Protein**: 13.4 g
- **Carbohydrates**: 12 g

Preparation Time: 10 minutes

Cooking Time: 15 minutes

Servings: 2

Ingredients:

- 1/3 cup cooked and diced chicken
- ½ cup cooked and chopped spinach
- 1/3 cup chopped artichokes
- 1 egg
- 1/3 cup (shredded) Mozzarella cheese
- 1 ounce cream cheese
- ¼ tsp. garlic powder

Directions:

1. Preheat a mini waffle maker if needed and grease it.
2. Incorporate all the ingredients.
3. Mix them all well.
4. Pour the mixture into the lower plate of the waffle maker and spread it evenly to cover the plate properly.
5. Close the lid.
6. Cook for at least 4 minutes to get the desired crunch.
7. Remove the chaffle from the heat and keep it aside for around one minute.
8. Make as many chaffles as your mixture and waffle maker allow.
9. Serve hot and enjoy!

Nutrition:

- **Calories:** 202
- **Fat:** 19 g
- **Protein:** 17 g
- **Carbohydrates:** 14 g

Preparation Time: 12 minutes

Cooking Time: 13 minutes

Servings: 2

Ingredients:

- 3-4 chicken pieces or ½ cup when done
- 1 tbsp. soy sauce
- 2 cloves garlic
- 1 cup cauliflower rice
- 2 eggs
- 1 cup Mozzarella cheese
- Salt to taste
- ¼ tsp. black pepper or to your taste
- ¼ tsp. white pepper or to your taste
- 1 stalk green onion

Directions:

1. Melt butter in oven or stove and set aside.
2. In a pot, cook the chicken by adding one cup of water to it with salt and bring it to a boil.
3. Seal the lid of the pot, then cook for 15–20 minutes.
4. When done, remove from stove and shred the chicken pieces leaving the bones behind; discard the bones.
5. Grate garlic finely into pieces.
6. In a small bowl, beat egg and mix chicken, garlic, cauliflower rice, soy sauce, black pepper, and white pepper.
7. Mix all the ingredients well.
8. Preheat the waffle maker if needed and grease it.
9. Place around 1/8 cup of shredded mozzarella cheese into the waffle maker.
10. Pour the mixture over the cheese on the waffle maker and add 1/8 cup shredded cheese on top as well.
11. Cook for 4–5 minutes or until it is done.
12. Repeat and make as many chaffles as the batter can.

13. Drizzle chopped green onion on top, then serve hot!

Nutrition:

- **Calories**: 288
- **Fat**: 11 g
- **Protein**: 19 g
- **Carbohydrates**: 11 g

Preparation Time: 15 minutes

Cooking Time: 10 minutes

Servings: 2

Ingredients:

For the Chaffle:

- 2 eggs
- 1 cup Mozzarella cheese (shredded)
- 1 tbsp. butter
- 2 tbsp. almond flour
- ¼ tsp. baking powder
- A pinch onion powder
- A pinch garlic powder
- A pinch salt

For the Chicken Patty:

- 1 lb. ground chicken
- ½ tbsp. onion powder
- ½ tbsp. garlic powder
- 1 cup Halloumi cheese
- ¼ tsp. salt or to your taste
- ¼ tsp. black pepper or to your taste

For Servings:

- 2 lettuce leaves
- 2 slices American cheese

Directions:

1. Mix all the chicken patty ingredients in a bowl.
2. Make equal-sized patties; either grill them or fry them.
3. Preheat a mini waffle maker if needed and grease it.
4. In a mixing bowl, add all the chaffle ingredients and mix well.

5. Pour the mixture to the lower plate of the waffle maker and spread it evenly to cover the plate properly, and close the lid

6. Cook for at least 4 minutes to get the desired crunch.

7. Remove the chaffle from the heat and keep it aside for around one minute.

8. Make as many chaffles as your mixture and waffle maker allow.

9. Serve with the chicken patties, lettuce, and a cheese slice in between two chaffles.

Nutrition:

- **Calories**: 219
- **Fat**: 21 g
- **Protein**: 16 g
- **Carbohydrates**: 17 g

Preparation Time: 15 minutes

Cooking Time: 25-30 minutes

Servings: 2

Ingredients:

For Chaffles:

- 2 eggs
- ½ cup Cheddar cheese
- 2 tbsp. Parmesan cheese
- ¼ tsp. Italian season
- 1 cup chicken

For Eggplant:

- 1 big eggplant
- 1 pinch salt
- 1 pinch black pepper

Directions:

1. Boil the chicken in water for 15 minutes and strain.
2. Shred the chicken into small pieces and set aside.
3. Cut the eggplant in slices and boil in water, and strain.
4. Add a pinch of salt and pepper.
5. Add all the chaffle ingredients to a bowl and mix well to make a mixture.
6. Add the boiled chicken as well.
7. Preheat a mini waffle maker if needed and grease it.
8. Pour the mixture into the lower plate of the waffle maker and spread it evenly to cover the plate properly.
9. Add the eggplant over two slices on the mixture and cover the lid.
10. Cook for at least 4 minutes to get the desired crunch.
11. Remove the chaffle from the heat and keep it aside for around one minute.
12. Make as many chaffles as your mixture and waffle maker allow.
13. Serve hot with your favorite sauce.

Nutrition:

- **Calories:** 299
- **Fat:** 20 g
- **Protein:** 15 g
- **Carbohydrates:** 13 g

Preparation Time: 20 minutes

Cooking Time: 10 minutes

Servings: 2

Ingredients:

- 1 cup chicken mince
- ¼ tsp. salt or to your taste
- ¼ tsp. black pepper or to your taste
- 2 eggs
- 1 tbsp. lemon juice
- 1 cup Mozzarella cheese (shredded)
- 2 tbsp. butter
- 1½ tsp. garlic powder
- ½ tsp. bay seasoning
- Parsley for garnishing

Directions:

1. In a frying pan, melt butter and add chicken mince.
2. When done, add salt, pepper, 1 tbsp. garlic powder, and lemon juice and put aside.
3. Whisk eggs and add mozzarella cheese to them with ½ garlic powder and bay seasoning.
4. Mix them all well and pour into the greasy mini waffle maker.
5. Cook for at least 4 minutes to get the desired crunch.
6. Remove the chaffle from the heat, add the chicken mixture in between, and fold.
7. Make as many chaffles as your mixture and waffle maker allow.
8. Top with parsley.
9. Serve hot and enjoy!

Nutrition:

- **Calories**: 255
- **Fat**: 24 g
- **Protein**: 19 g
- **Carbohydrates**: 12 g

Preparation Time: 25 minutes

Cooking Time: 17 minutes

Servings: 2

Ingredients:

For Chaffle:

- 1 egg
- ½ cup Mozzarella cheese (shredded)

For Fried Chicken:

- 8 pieces chicken strips
- 2 tbsp. butter
- ¼ tsp. salt or to your taste
- ¼ tsp. black pepper or to your taste
- ½ tsp. red chili flakes

Directions:

1. In a frying pan, melt butter and fry chicken strips on medium-low heat.
2. Add the spices at the end and set them aside.
3. Mix all the chaffle ingredients.
4. Fill in a thin layer on a prepared waffle iron.
5. Stir in chicken strips and pour more mixture again over the top.
6. Cook the chaffle for around 5 minutes.
7. Make as many chaffles as your mixture and waffle maker allow.
8. Serve hot!

Nutrition:

- **Calories:** 262
- **Fat:** 26 g
- **Protein:** 19 g
- **Carbohydrates:** 12 g

Preparation Time: 15 minutes

Cooking Time: 7 minutes

Servings: 2

Ingredients:

For Garlic Chicken:

- 1 cup chicken mince
- ¼ tsp. salt or to your taste
- ¼ tsp. black pepper or to your taste
- 1 tbsp. lemon juice
- 2 tbsp. butter
- 2 tbsp. garlic juvenile
- 1 tsp. garlic powder
- 1 tbsp. soy sauce

For Chaffle:

- 2 eggs
- 1 cup Mozzarella cheese (shredded)
- 1 tsp. garlic powder

For Servings:

- ½ cup (diced) cucumber
- 1 tbsp. parsley

Directions:

1. In a frying pan, melt butter and add juvenile garlic and sauté for 1 minute.
2. Now add chicken mince and cook till it tenders.
3. When done, add the rest of the ingredients. Keep aside.
4. Whisk eggs and add mozzarella cheese to them with garlic powder.
5. Mix them all well and pour into the greasy mini waffle maker.
6. Cook for at least 4 minutes to get the desired crunch.
7. Remove the chaffle from the heat, add the chicken mixture in between with cucumber, and fold.
8. Make as many chaffles as your mixture and waffle maker allow.

9. Serve hot and top with parsley.

Nutrition:

- **Calories**: 277
- **Fat**: 19 g
- **Protein**: 11 g
- **Carbohydrates**: 13 g

Preparation Time: 15 minutes

Cooking Time: 7 minutes

Servings: 2

Ingredients:

For the Chaffle:

- 2 eggs
- 1 cup Mozzarella cheese (shredded)
- 1 tbsp. butter
- 2 tbsp. almond flour
- ¼ tsp. baking powder
- A pinch salt

For the Chicken:

- 2-4 chicken pieces
- ½ tbsp. ginger powder
- ¼ tsp. salt or to your taste
- ¼ tsp. black pepper or to your taste
- 1 tbsp. soy sauce
- 1 stalk spring onion

Directions:

1. Boil the chicken in a saucepan, when done remove from water, and pat dry.
2. Shred the chicken into small pieces and add all the seasoning and spices.
3. Thinly chop the spring onion and mix with the chicken, and set aside.
4. Preheat a mini waffle maker if needed and grease it.
5. In a mixing bowl, add all the chaffle ingredients and mix well.
6. Pour a little amount of mixture into the lower plate of the waffle maker and spread it evenly. to cover the plate properly
7. Add the chicken mixture on top and again spread the thin layer of mixture and close the lid.
8. Cook for at least 4 minutes to get the desired crunch.
9. Remove the chaffle from the heat.

10. Make as many chaffles as your mixture and waffle maker allow.

11. Serve hot and enjoy.

Nutrition:

- **Calories**: 247
- **Fat**: 14 g
- **Protein**: 9 g
- **Carbohydrates**: 10 g

Preparation Time: 15 minutes

Cooking Time: 7 minutes

Servings: 2

Ingredients:

- 2 eggs
- 1½ cup Cheddar cheese
- 16 slices Deli jalapeno
- 1 cup boiled chicken (shredded)

Directions:

1. Preheat a mini waffle maker if needed.
2. Whisk eggs and add chicken and half cheddar cheese to them.
3. Mix them all well
4. Shred some of the remaining cheddar cheese to the lower plate of the waffle maker.
5. Now pour the mixture into the shredded cheese.
6. Add the cheese again on the top with around 4 slices of jalapeno and close the lid.
7. Cook for at least 4 minutes to get the desired crunch.
8. Serve hot.
9. Make as many chaffles as your mixture allows.

Nutrition:

- **Calories:** 302
- **Fat:** 26 g
- **Protein:** 13.4 g
- **Carbohydrates:** 14 g

Preparation Time: 25 minutes

Cooking Time: 17 minutes

Servings: 2

Ingredients:

For Chaffle:

- 2 eggs
- ½ cup Mozzarella cheese (shredded)
- ¼ tsp. garlic powder
- ¼ tsp. salt or to your taste
- ¼ tsp. black pepper or to your taste

For Stuffing:

- 1 small diced onion
- 1 cup chicken
- 4 tbsp. butter
- ¼ tsp. salt or to your taste
- ¼ tsp. black pepper or to your taste

Directions:

1. Preheat a mini waffle maker if needed and grease it
2. In a mixing bowl, add all the chaffle ingredients
3. Mix them all well
4. Pour the mixture to the lower plate of the waffle maker and spread it evenly to cover the plate properly, and close the lid
5. Cook for at least 4 minutes to get the desired crunch
6. Remove the chaffle from the heat and keep it aside
7. Make as many chaffles as your mixture and waffle maker allow
8. Using a small frying pan, cook butter in it on medium-low heat
9. Sauté chicken and onion and add salt and pepper
10. Take another bowl and tear chaffles down into minute pieces
11. Add chicken and onion to it

12. Take a casserole dish, and add this new stuffing mixture to it

13. Bake at 350F for 32 minutes and serve hot

Nutrition:

- **Calories**: 284
- **Fat**: 16 g
- **Protein**: 13.4 g
- **Carbohydrates**: 10 g

Preparation Time: 15 minutes

Cooking Time: 7 minutes

Servings: 2

Ingredients:

For the Chaffle:

- 2 eggs
- 1 cup Mozzarella cheese (shredded)
- A pinch salt

For the Chicken:

- 2-4 chicken pieces
- ½ tbsp. ginger powder
- ¼ tsp. salt or to your taste
- ¼ tsp. black pepper or as per your taste
- 3 tbsp. cauliflower
- 3 tbsp. cabbage
- 1 tbsp. green pepper
- 1 stalk spring onion

Directions:

1. Boil the chicken, green pepper, cauliflower, and cabbage in a saucepan; when done strain the water.
2. Shred the chicken into small pieces and blend all the vegetables and mix them together.
3. Thinly chop the spring onion and stir with the chicken, and set aside.
4. Preheat a mini waffle maker if needed and grease it.
5. In a mixing bowl, add all the chaffle ingredients and mix well.
6. Pour a little amount of mixture into the lower plate of the waffle maker and spread it evenly to cover the plate properly.
7. Add the chicken mixture on top and again spread the thin layer of mixture and close the lid.
8. Cook for at least 4 minutes to get the desired crunch.
9. Remove the chaffle from the heat.

10. Make as many chaffles as your mixture and waffle maker allow.

11. Serve hot and enjoy.

Nutrition:

- **Calories**: 292
- **Fat**: 26 g
- **Protein**: 13.4 g
- **Carbohydrates**: 10 g

Preparation Time: 15 minutes

Cooking Time: 7 minutes

Servings: 2

Ingredients:

- 3–4 pieces chicken or ½ cup when done
- 1 tbsp. soy sauce
- 2 cloves garlic
- 1 cup cabbage
- 2 eggs
- 1 cup Mozzarella cheese
- Salt to your taste
- ¼ tsp. black pepper or as per your taste
- ¼ tsp. white pepper or to your taste

Directions:

1. Melt butter in oven or stove and set aside.
2. In a pot, cook the chicken and cabbage by adding one cup of water to it with salt and bring to boil.
3. Seal the lid of the pot, then cook for 15–20 minutes.
4. When done, remove from stove and shred the chicken pieces leaving the bones behind; discard the bones.
5. Strain water from cabbage and blend.
6. Grate garlic finely into pieces.
7. In a small bowl, beat egg and mix chicken, cabbage, garlic, soy sauce, black pepper, and white pepper.
8. Mix all the ingredients well.
9. Preheat the waffle maker if needed and grease it.
10. Place around 1/8 cup of shredded mozzarella cheese into the waffle maker.
11. Pour the mixture over the cheese on the waffle maker and add 1/8 cup shredded cheese on top as well.
12. Cook for 4–5 minutes or until it is done.

13. Make as many chaffles as your mixture and waffle maker allow.

14. Serve hot!

Nutrition:

- **Calories**: 294
- **Fat**: 36 g
- **Protein**: 21 g
- **Carbohydrates**: 20 g

189. CHICKEN ZUCCHINI CHAFFLE

Preparation Time: 15 minutes

Cooking Time: 7 minutes

Servings: 2

Ingredients:

- 1 cup chicken boneless pieces
- 1 zucchini (small)
- 2 eggs
- Salt to your taste
- 1 cup Shredded mozzarella
- 2 tbsp. Parmesan
- Pepper to your taste
- 1 tsp. basil
- ½ cup water

Directions:

1. In a small saucepan, add chicken with a half cup of water and boil till chicken tenders.
2. Preheat your waffle iron.
3. Grate zucchini finely.
4. Add all the ingredients to zucchini in a bowl and mix well.
5. Shred chicken finely and add it as well.
6. Grease your waffle iron lightly.
7. Pour the mixture into a full-size waffle maker and spread evenly.
8. Cook till it turns crispy.
9. Make as many chaffles as your mixture and waffle maker allow.
10. Serve crispy and hot.

Nutrition:

- **Calories**: 299
- **Fat**: 16 g
- **Protein**: 23.4 g
- **Carbohydrates**: 14 g

Preparation Time: 25 minutes

Cooking Time: 17 minutes

Servings: 2

Ingredients:

- ½ cup spinach
- ½ cup boneless chicken
- 1 egg
- 1/2 cup shredded mozzarella
- Pepper to your taste
- 1 tbsp. garlic powder
- 1 tbsp. onion powder
- Salt to your taste
- 1 tsp. basil

Directions:

1. Boil chicken in water to make it tender.
2. Shred-it into small pieces and set aside.
3. Boil spinach in a saucepan for 10 minutes and strain.
4. Preheat your waffle iron.
5. Add all the ingredients to boiled spinach in a bowl and mix well.
6. Now add the shredded chicken.
7. Grease your waffle iron lightly.
8. Pour the mixture into a full-size waffle maker and spread evenly.
9. Cook till it turns crispy.
10. Make as many chaffles as your mixture and waffle maker allow.
11. Serve crispy and with your favorite keto sauce.

Nutrition:

- **Calories:** 292
- **Fat:** 26 g
- **Protein:** 14 g
- **Carbohydrates:** 18 g

Preparation Time: 15 minutes

Cooking Time: 17 minutes

Servings: 2

Ingredients:

- ½ cup chicken
- 1 tbsp. butter
- 1 tbsp. BBQ sauce (sugar-free)
- 2 tbsp. almond flour
- 1 egg
- ½ cup Cheddar cheese

Directions:

1. Cook the chicken in the butter on low-medium heat for 10 minutes.
2. Preheat your waffle iron.
3. In a mixing bowl, add all the chaffle ingredients, including chicken, and mix well
4. Grease your waffle iron lightly.
5. Pour the mixture to the bottom plate evenly; also spread it out to get better results and close the upper plate, and heat.
6. Cook for 6 minutes or until the chaffle is done.
7. Make as many chaffles as your mixture and waffle maker allow.

Nutrition:

- **Calories:** 257
- **Fat:** 26 g
- **Protein:** 13.4 g
- **Carbohydrates:** 18 g

Preparation Time: 5 minutes

Cooking Time: 5 minutes

Servings: 2

Ingredients:

- 15 oz. 1 packet tuna
- ½ cup mozzarella cheese
- 1 egg
- Pinch salt

Directions:

1. In a small bowl, preheat the mini waffle maker, add the egg, and whip it.
2. Stir in the fish, butter, and salt and combine well.
3. Add a tsp. of cheese to the mini waffle maker for about 30 seconds before adding the formula's mixture. When the tuna chaffle is cooked, this will allow the cheese to get crispy. This is the form I use!
4. Attach ½ of the waffle maker mixture and cook for at least 4 minutes.
5. Cut it and cook another 4 minutes of the last tuna chaffle.

Nutrition:

- **Calories**: 292
- **Fat**: 26 g
- **Protein**: 29 g
- **Carbohydrates**: 18 g

Preparation Time: 15 minutes

Cooking Time: 15 minutes

Servings: 4

Ingredients:

- 1 lb. cod fillets, sliced into 4 slices
- 1 tsp. sea salt
- 1 tsp. garlic powder
- 1 egg, whisked
- 1 cup almond flour
- 2 tbsp. avocado oil

Chaffle Ingredients:

- 2 eggs
- ½ cup cheddar cheese
- 2 tbsps. almond flour
- ½ tsp. Italian seasoning

Directions:

1. Mix together the chaffle ingredients in a bowl and make 4 square.
2. Put the chaffles in a preheated chaffle maker.
3. Mix together the salt, pepper, and garlic powder in a mixing bowl. Toss the cod cubes in this mixture and let sit for 10 minutes.
4. Then dip each cod slice into the egg mixture and then into the almond flour.
5. Heat oil in skillet and fish cubes for about 2–3 minutes, until cooked and browned
6. Serve on chaffles and enjoy!

Nutrition:

- **Calories:** 252
- **Fat:** 21 g
- **Protein:** 11 g
- **Carbohydrates:** 18 g

Preparation Time: 15 minutes

Cooking Time: 10 minutes

Servings: 2

Ingredients:

For Chaffle:

- 2 eggs
- 1 cup Mozzarella cheese (shredded)
- ½ tsp. bay seasoning
- ¼ tsp. garlic powder

For Fried Fish:

- 1 cup fish boneless
- 1 tbsp. garlic powder
- 1 tbsp. onion powder
- ¼ tsp. salt or to your taste
- ¼ tsp. black pepper or to your taste
- ¼ tsp. turmeric:
- ½ tbsp. red chili flakes:
- 2 tbsp. butter

Directions:

1. Marinate the fish with all the ingredients of the fried fish except for butter.
2. Melt butter in a medium-size frying pan and add the marinated fish.
3. Fry from both sides for at least 5 minutes and set aside.
4. Preheat a mini waffle maker if needed and grease it.
5. Whisk eggs and add all the chaffle ingredients.
6. Mix them all well.
7. Pour the mixture into the lower plate of the waffle maker and spread it evenly to cover the plate properly.
8. Close the lid.
9. Cook for at least 4 minutes to get the desired crunch.

10. Remove the chaffle from the heat and keep it aside for around one minute.

11. Make as many chaffles as your mixture and waffle maker allow.

12. Serve hot with the prepared fish.

Nutrition:

- **Calories**: 261
- **Fat**: 22 g
- **Protein**: 13 g
- **Carbohydrates**: 17 g

Preparation Time: 25 minutes

Cooking Time: 10 minutes

Servings: 2

Ingredients:

For Chaffle:

- 1 egg
- ½ cup Mozzarella cheese (shredded)
- ¼ tsp. salt or to your taste
- ¼ tsp. black pepper or as per your taste
- 1 tbsp. ginger powder:

For Crab:

- 1 cup crab meat
- 2 tbsp. butter
- ¼ tsp. salt or to your taste
- ¼ tsp. black pepper or as per your taste
- ½ tsp. red chili flakes:

Directions:

1. In a frying pan, melt butter and fry crab meat for two minutes.
2. Add the spices at the end and set them aside.
3. Mix all the chaffle ingredients.
4. Fill in a thin layer on a preheated waffle iron.
5. Stir in prepared crab and pour more mixture again over the top.
6. Cook the chaffle for around 5 minutes.
7. Make as many chaffles as your mixture and waffle maker allow.
8. Serve hot with your favorite sauce.

Nutrition:

- **Calories:** 262
- **Fat:** 20 g
- **Protein:** 10 g
- **Carbohydrates:** 8 g

Preparation Time: 15 minutes

Cooking Time: 27 minutes

Servings: 2

Ingredients:

Fish Cakes:

- 9 ounces (249 g) raw cod, skinless and boneless
- 1 large egg
- 1 clove garlic, minced
- 2 tbsp. coconut flour
- 2 tsp. curry powder
- 1 tsp. red pepper flakes
- ½ tsp. ground cumin
- ½ tsp. paprika
- ¼ tsp. salt
- Pinch black pepper
- 1 medium spring onion, chopped
- 1 tbsp. chopped fresh cilantro
- 2 tsp. ghee

Sriracha Mayonnaise:

- 2 tbsp. mayonnaise
- 2 tsp. Sriracha sauce

Topping:

- 2 to 4 lettuce leaves

Directions:

1. Prepare a batch of the Basic Savory Chaffles by following the instructions of the first recipe. When done, set aside.
2. Place all the ingredients, except for the spring onion, cilantro, and ghee, in a blender. Process until smooth. Add the spring onion and cilantro and stir through.
3. Make the patties: Place the fish mixture in a mixing bowl. Form the mixture into 2 large fish cakes.

4. Preheat a big pan greased with the ghee over medium heat. When hot, stir in the patties and cook for 5 to 7 minutes per side or until crisp. Use a spatula to flip them over. Set the cooked patties aside.

5. Meanwhile, prepare the dressing by simply combining the mayonnaise and Sriracha. Set aside.

6. Place the lettuce on both chaffles. Top with the spicy fish patties and drizzle with the prepared Sriracha mayonnaise. Serve warm.

Nutrition:

- **Calories**: 535
- **Fat**: 36.6 g
- **Protein**: 40.7 g
- **Carbohydrates**: 29 g

Preparation Time: 15 minutes

Cooking Time: 10 minutes

Servings: 2

Ingredients:

- 1 egg, lightly beaten
- ½ cup cheddar cheese, shredded
- 16 oz. canned tuna

Directions:

1. Prepare your waffle maker.
2. Whisk egg, cheese, tuna, and salt until combined.
3. Fill in half of the batter in the hot waffle maker and cook for 4 minutes. Repeat with the remaining batter.
4. Serve and enjoy.

Nutrition:

- **Calories:** 261
- **Fat:** 23 g
- **Protein:** 19 g
- **Carbohydrates:** 16 g

Preparation Time: 10 minutes

Cooking Time: 25 minutes

Servings: 6

Ingredients:

- 1 lb. crab meat
- 1/3 cup Panko breadcrumbs
- 1 egg
- 2 tbsp. fat Greek yogurt
- 1 tsp. Dijon mustard
- 2 tbsp. parsley and chives, fresh
- 1 tsp. Italian seasoning
- 1 lemon, juiced
- Salt, pepper to taste

Directions:

1. Preheat the waffle maker.
2. Incorporate all the ingredients, except crab meat.
3. Add the meat. Mix well.
4. Form the mixture into round patties.
5. Cook 1 patty for 3 minutes.
6. Remove it and repeat the process with the remaining crab chaffle mixture.
7. Once ready, remove and enjoy warm.

Nutrition:

- **Calories**: 263
- **Fat**: 25 g
- **Protein**: 14 g
- **Carbohydrates**: 16 g

Preparation Time: 15 minutes

Cooking Time: 15 minutes

Servings: 1

Chaffle Ingredients:

- Classic Chaffle Recipe

Japanese Toppings Ingredients:

- 1 whole avocado, ripe
- 5 slices pickled ginger
- 1 tbsp. gluten-free soy sauce
- 1/3 cup edamame
- ¼ cup Japanese pickled vegetables
- ½ pound sushi-grade salmon, sliced
- ¼ tsp. wasabi

Directions:

1. Cut the salmon and avocado into thin slices. Set aside.
2. If the edamame is frozen, boil it in a pot of water until done. Set aside.
3. Follow the Classic Chaffle recipe.
4. Once the chaffles are done, pour a tbsp. of soy sauce onto the chaffle and then layer the salmon, avocado, edamame, pickled ginger, pickled vegetables, and wasabi.
5. Enjoy!

Nutrition:

- **Calories**: 264
- **Fat**: 27 g
- **Protein**: 14 g
- **Carbohydrates**: 13 g

Preparation Time: 15 minutes

Cooking Time: 15 minutes

Servings: 1

Chaffle ingredients

- Classic Chaffle Recipe or Sweet Chaffle Recipe
- 2 tbsps. Everything Bagel Seasoning

Filling Ingredients:
- 1 ounce cream cheese
- 1 beefsteak tomato, thinly sliced
- 4–6 ounces salmon gravlax
- 1 small shallot, thinly sliced
- capers
- 1 tbsp. fresh dill

Directions:

1. Slice the tomato and the shallots.
2. Follow the Classic Chaffle recipe and add bagel seasoning.
3. Once the chaffles are done, sprinkle more everything bagel seasoning onto the tops of both chaffles.
4. Lay two chaffles side by side and layer on the cream cheese, salmon, and shallots.
5. Sprinkle dill and capers and sandwich the two chaffles together.
6. Enjoy!

Nutrition:

- **Calories**: 272
- **Fat**: 21 g
- **Protein**: 11 g
- **Carbohydrates**: 10 g

Preparation Time: 10 minutes

Cooking Time: 5 minutes

Servings: 1

Ingredients:

- 1 large egg
- ¼ cup cheddar cheese, shredded
- 1 tbsp. almond flour
- ¼ tsp. baking powder
- ½ tsp. garlic powder
- 1 tbsp. minced parsley

For Serving:

- 1 poach egg
- 4 oz. smoked salmon

Directions:

1. Preheat your dash mini waffle maker and let it heat up and grease with cooking spray.
2. Mix together egg, cheese, almond flour, baking powder, garlic powder, parsley to a mixing bowl until combined well.
3. Pour batter in-dash mini waffle maker.
4. Close the lid.
5. Cook chaffles for about 2–3 minutes or until cooked or no soggy.
6. Serve chaffles on the plate with smoked salmon and poach the egg.

Nutrition:

- **Calories:** 267
- **Fat:** 21 g
- **Protein:** 12 g
- **Carbohydrates:** 19 g

Preparation Time: 45 minutes

Cooking Time: 30 minutes

Servings: 3

Ingredients:

- 1 egg
- ½ cup shredded cheddar cheese
- 1 tbsp. almond flour
- 2 tsp. Cajun seasoning
- 1 lb. raw shrimp
- 1 tbsp. avocado oil
- 2 slices bacon
- 1/3 cup sliced red onions

Directions:

1. This sandwich is full of nutrients and contains a lot of ingredients. So let's start by preparing the ingredients. To begin with, heating a pan to medium heat with avocado oil. Then add the bacon strips to the pan and let each side cook until crispy and brown.
2. Remove the bacon strips and dry them on a paper towel. This will help absorb excess oil.
3. Then prepare the shrimps. Put them in a bowl and add 1 tsp. of Cajun seasoning. Add a small amount of avocado oil and salt and pepper. Leave them for 15 minutes.
4. Then put the shrimps in the pan and fry them in the same bacon grease. Fry each side for a small amount of time. Once they are fried, dry them on kitchen paper. Scoop out the avocado in a bowl.
5. Then prepare your chaffle bread. For the chaffle bread, add an egg with shredded cheddar cheese, almond flour, 1 tsp. of Cajun seasoning and cook in waffle machine that is preheated to medium heat for around 3 to 4 minutes.
6. Then assemble your Cajun Shrimp and Avocado chaffle sandwich. Add the shrimps, onions, bacon slices, and avocado. Then your scrumptious sandwich will be ready.

Nutrition:

- **Calories**: 390
- **Protein**: 19 g
- **Fat**: 16 g
- **Carbohydrates**: 14 g

Preparation Time: 15 minutes

Cooking Time: 31 minutes

Servings: 4

Ingredients:

For the Shrimp:

- 1 tbsp. olive oil
- 1 lb. jumbo shrimp, peeled and deveined
- 1 tbsp. Creole seasoning
- Salt to taste
- 2 tbsp. hot sauce
- 3 tbsp. butter
- 2 tbsp. chopped fresh scallions to garnish

For the Chaffles:

- 2 eggs, beaten
- 1 cup finely grated Monterey Jack cheese

Directions:

For the Shrimp:

1. Cook olive oil in a medium skillet over medium heat.
2. Season the shrimp with the Creole seasoning and salt. Cook in the oil until pink and opaque on both sides, 2 minutes.
3. Pour in the hot sauce and butter. Mix well until the shrimp is adequately coated in the sauce, 1 minute.
4. Turn the heat off and set aside.

For the Chaffles:

1. Preheat the waffle iron.
2. Beat eggs and Monterey Jack cheese.
3. Open the iron and add a quarter of the mixture. Close and cook until crispy, 7 minutes.
4. Transfer the chaffle to a plate and make 3 more chaffles in the same manner.
5. Cut the chaffles into quarters and place them on a plate.
6. Garnish with the scallions.

7. Serve warm.

Nutrition:

- **Calories**: 267
- **Fat**: 29 g
- **Protein**: 14 g
- **Carbohydrates**: 10 g

Preparation Time: 10 minutes

Cooking Time: 32 minutes

Servings: 4

Ingredients:

- 2 cups shredded mozzarella cheese
- 4 large eggs
- ½ tsp. curry powder
- ½ tsp. oregano
- Shrimp Sandwich Filling:
- 1-pound raw shrimp (peeled and deveined)
- 1 large avocado (diced)
- 4 slices cooked bacon
- 2 tbsp. sour cream
- ½ tsp. paprika
- 1 tsp. Cajun seasoning
- 1 tbsp. olive oil
- ¼ cup onion (finely chopped)
- 1 red bell pepper (diced)

Directions:

1. Plug the waffle maker to preheat it and spray it with a non-stick cooking spray.
2. Beat the eggs into a mixing bowl and beat. Add the cheese, oregano, and curry. Mix until the ingredients are well combined.
3. Pour an appropriate amount of the batter into the waffle maker and spread out the batter to the edges to cover all the holes on the waffle maker. This should make 8 mini waffles.
4. Seal the waffle maker, then cook for about 4 minutes or according to your waffle maker's settings.
5. After the cooking cycle, use a silicone or plastic utensil to remove the chaffle from the waffle maker.
6. Do step 3 to 5 until you have cooked all the batter into chaffles.
7. Cook the olive oil in a big skillet over medium to high heat.

8. Add the shrimp and cook until the shrimp is pink and tender.

9. Remove the skillet from heat and use a slotted spoon to transfer the shrimp to a paper towel-lined plate to drain for a few minutes.

10. Put the shrimp in a mixing bowl. Add paprika and Cajun seasoning. Toss until the shrimps are all coated with seasoning.

11. To assemble the sandwich, place one chaffle on a flat surface and spread some sour cream over it. Layer some shrimp, onion, avocado, diced pepper, and one slice of bacon over it. Cover with another chaffle.

12. Repeat step 10 until you have assembled all the ingredients into sandwiches.

13. Serve and enjoy.

Nutrition:

- **Calories**: 277
- **Fat**: 29 g
- **Protein**: 19 g
- **Carbohydrates**: 16 g

Preparation Time: 5 minutes

Cooking Time: 10 minutes

Servings: 3

Ingredients:

- 1 large egg
- 1 tbsp. almond flour
- 1 tbsp. full-fat Greek yogurt
- 1/8 tsp. baking powder
- ¼ cup shredded Swiss cheese

Topping:

- 4oz. grill prawns
- 4 oz. steamed cauliflower mash
- ½ zucchini sliced
- 3 lettuce leaves
- 1 tomato, sliced
- 1 tbsp. flax seeds

Directions:

1. Make 3 chaffles with the given chaffles ingredients.
2. For serving, arrange lettuce leaves on each chaffle.
3. Top with zucchini slice, grill prawns, cauliflower mash, and a tomato slice.
4. Drizzle flax seeds on top.
5. Serve and enjoy!

Nutrition:

- **Calories:** 266
- **Fat:** 24 g
- **Protein:** 19 g
- **Carbohydrates:** 10 g

Preparation Time: 10 minutes

Cooking Time: 10 minutes

Servings: 2

Ingredients:

- 1 large egg
- ½ cup shredded mozzarella
- 1 tbsp. cream cheese
- 2 slices salmon
- 1 tbsp. everything bagel seasoning

Directions:

1. Turn on the waffle maker to heat and oil it with cooking spray.
2. Beat egg in a bowl, then add ½ cup mozzarella.
3. Pour half of the mixture into the waffle maker and cook for 3-4 minutes.
4. Remove and repeat with the remaining mixture.
5. Let chaffles cool, then spread cream cheese, sprinkle with seasoning, and top with salmon.

Nutrition:

- **Calories:** 201
- **Fat:** 1 g
- **Protein:** 5 g
- **Carbohydrates:** 9 g

Preparation Time: 15 minutes

Cooking Time: 10 minutes

Servings: 2

Ingredients:

Cajun Aromatized Chaffle:

- 4 eggs, should be large
- 2 cups shredded mozzarella part-skim cheese
- 1 tsp. Seasoning Cajun

Filling for Sandwich

- 1-pound fresh shrimp peeled and deveined
- 1 tbsp. bacon (or avocado) grease
- 4 slices bacon cooked
- 1 large sliced avocado
- ¼ cup red onion, thinly sliced
- 1 dish bacon scallion cream cheese spread optional
- 1 tsp. Seasoning (Cajun)

Directions:

1. Whisk the eggs together. Add 2 cups of mozzarella cheese with low moisture and 1 tsp. of Cajun seasoning. Put ¼ cup of cheese and a mixture of eggs over a mini waffle pan. Cook until the chaffle is browned. Repeat the process with the left egg and cheese batter
2. Add shrimp and combine it in a large bowl, with the remaining 1 tsp. of Cajun seasoning. Garnish with salt and pepper. Fried in a pan over medium-high heat with bacon grease until the shrimp is translucent. Lift the fried shrimp and put aside. Let cool if desired
3. Place bacon scallion cream cheese over a side of a chaffle to create the Chaffle Sandwich: cover the top of the chaffle with shrimp, bacon, avocado, and red onion. Cover with one more chaffle. Serve as you wish

Nutrition:

- **Calories:** 488
- **Fat:** 32.22 g
- **Protein:** 47.59 g
- **Carbohydrates:** 22 g

Preparation Time: 20 minutes

Cooking Time: 5 minutes

Servings: 1-2

Ingredients:

- 1 egg
- 3/4 cup almond flour
- ½ tsp. baking powder
- 1/8 t salt
- 2 tbsp. melted butter
- ¼ cup mozzarella shredded cheese
- ¼ cup sour cream

Directions:

1. Mix together the ingredients and place the batter into a mini waffle iron to produce a batch of chaffles.
2. Tuna Sandwich: Take two chaffles and bring them together to make a sandwich with your St. Jude tuna salad. Choose your unique flavor of St. Jude tuna: blend with a little bit of olive oil and pepper. Add pepperoncini, tomatoes, red onion, red peppers, and all other preferred toppings.

Nutrition:

- **Calories**: 100
- **Fat**: 37 g
- **Protein**: 96 g
- **Carbohydrates**: 29 g

Preparation Time: 15 minutes

Cooking Time: 28 minutes

Servings: 2

Ingredients:

Salmon Patties:

- Ounces (249 g) canned salmon
- 1 large egg
- ¼ cup almond flour
- 1 tbsp. chopped fresh dill
- 1 small spring onion, chopped
- 1 clove garlic, minced
- ½ tsp. paprika
- ¼ tsp. salt
- Pinch black pepper
- 2 tsp. ghee

Lemon Dressing:

- 3 tbsp. mayonnaise
- 1½ tsp. fresh lemon juice
- ½ tsp. fresh lemon zest
- 1 tsp. extra-virgin olive oil
- ¼ tsp. Dijon mustard
- Salt and pepper, to taste
- 1 tsp. chopped fresh parsley

Topping:

- 2 to 4 lettuce leaves

Directions:

1. Prepare a batch of the Basic Savory Chaffles by following the instructions of the first recipe. When done, set aside.

2. Make the patties. Stir together all the ingredients for the salmon patties, except for the ghee, in a mixing bowl. Form the mixture into 2 large fish cakes.

3. Preheat a big pan greased with the ghee over medium heat. When hot, stir in the patties and cook for 5 to 7 minutes per side or until crisp. Use a spatula to flip them over. Set the cooked patties aside.

4. Meanwhile, prepare the lemon dressing by combining the mayonnaise, lemon juice, lemon zest, olive oil, Dijon mustard, salt, pepper, and parsley in another bowl. Set aside.

5. Top the chaffles with lettuce and salmon patties. Drizzle with the prepared dressing and top with the remaining chaffles.

6. Serve warm.

Nutrition:

- **Calories**: 952
- **Fat**: 74.2 g
- **Protein**: 64.3 g
- **Carbohydrates**: 56 g

Preparation Time: 10 minutes

Cooking Time: 5 minutes

Servings: 1

Ingredients:

- ½ cup canned tuna, drained
- 1½ tbsp. mayonnaise
- 1 tsp. fresh lemon juice
- ¼ tsp. Dijon mustard
- 1 small spring onion, chopped
- Salt and ground black pepper, to taste
- 2 slices provolone cheese

Directions:

1. Follow the instructions of the first recipe for the Basic Chaffles with a mini waffle maker. When the chaffles are done, allow them to cool on a cooling rack and set aside.
2. In a bowl, combine the tuna, mayonnaise, lemon juice, Dijon mustard, and spring onion. Season with salt and pepper to taste.
3. Spoon the tuna filling on top of one chaffle. Top with the slices of cheese. Top with the other chaffle. Serve immediately.

Nutrition:

- **Calories:** 827
- **Fat:** 66.9 g
- **Protein:** 50.3 g
- **Carbohydrates:** 42 g

211. Cheesy Salmon Chaffles

Preparation Time: 5 minutes

Cooking Time: 7 minutes

Servings: 2

Ingredients:

- 2 Basic Savory Chaffles
- ¼ cup cream cheese
- 2 to 3 slices smoked salmon
- 1 tbsp. chopped chives
- Pinch black pepper

Directions:

1. Prepare a batch of the Basic Savory Chaffles by following the instructions of the first recipe.
2. Let the chaffles cool down and spread the cream cheese and smoked salmon on top. Sprinkle with chives and black pepper.
3. Serve immediately.

Nutrition:

- **Calories**: 332
- **Fat**: 28.1 g
- **Protein**: 19.7 g
- **Carbohydrates**: 16 g

Preparation Time: 10 minutes

Cooking Time: 10 minutes

Servings: 2

Ingredients:

- 1 chicken breasts cut into 2x2 inch chunks
- 1 egg, whisked
- ¼ cup almond flour
- 2 tbsps. onion powder
- 2 tbsps. garlic powder
- 1 tsp. dried oregano
- 1 tsp. paprika powder
- 1 tsp. salt
- ½ tsp. black pepper
- 2 tbsps. avocado oil

Directions:

1. Add all the dry ingredients together into a large bowl. Mix well.
2. Place the eggs into a separate bowl.
3. Dip each chicken piece into the egg and then into the dry ingredients.
4. Heat oil in 10-inch skillet, add oil.
5. Once avocado oil is hot, place the coated chicken nuggets onto a skillet and cook for 6-8 minutes until cooked and golden brown.
6. Serve with chaffles and raspberries.
7. Enjoy!

Nutrition:

- **Calories:** 401
- **Fat:** 219 g
- **Protein:** 32.35 g
- **Carbohydrates:** 3 g

Preparation Time: 10 minutes

Cooking Time: 15 minutes

Servings: 2

Ingredients:

- 1 lb. cod fillets, sliced into 4 slices
- 1 tsp. sea salt
- 1 tsp. garlic powder
- 1 egg, whisked
- 1 cup almond flour
- 2 tbsp. avocado oil

Chaffle Ingredients:

- 2 eggs
- ½ cup cheddar cheese
- 2 tbsps. almond flour
- ½ tsp. Italian seasoning

Directions:

1. Mix together chaffle ingredients in a bowl and make 4 squares
2. Put the chaffles in a preheated chaffle maker.
3. Mix together the salt, pepper, and garlic powder in a mixing bowl. Toss the cod cubes in this mixture and let sit for 10 minutes.
4. Then dip each cod slice into the egg mixture and then into the almond flour.
5. Heat oil in skillet and fish cubes for about 2–3 minutes, until cooked and browned
6. Serve on chaffles and enjoy!

Nutrition:

- **Calories:** 121
- **Fat:** 59 g
- **Protein:** 38 g
- **Carbohydrates:** 3 g

Preparation Time: 10 minutes

Cooking Time: 15 minutes

Servings: 2

Ingredients:

- ½ cup mozzarella, shredded
- 1 egg
- I pinch garlic powder

Pork Patty:

- ½ cup pork, minutes
- 1 tbsp. green onion, diced
- ½ tsp. Italian seasoning
- Lettuce leaves

Directions:

1. Preheat the square waffle maker and grease with.
2. Mix together egg, cheese, and garlic powder in a small mixing bowl.
3. Pour batter into a preheated waffle maker and close the lid.
4. Make 2 chaffles from this batter.
5. Cook chaffles for about 2–3 minutes, until cooked through.
6. Meanwhile, mix together pork patty ingredients in a bowl and make 1 large patty.
7. Grill pork patty in a preheated grill for about 3–4 minutes per side until cooked through.
8. Arrange pork patty between two chaffles with lettuce leaves. Cut sandwich to make a triangular sandwich.
9. Enjoy!

Nutrition:

- **Calories:** 26
- **Protein:** 48 g
- **Fat:** 48 g
- **Carbohydrates:** 4 g

Preparation Time: 10 minutes

Cooking Time: 15 Minutes

Servings: 2

Ingredients:

- 1 large egg
- ½ cup jack cheese, shredded
- 1 pinch salt

For Serving:

- 1 chicken leg
- Salt
- Pepper to taste
- 1 tsp. garlic, minutes
- 1 egg
- 1 tsp. avocado oil

Directions:

1. Heat your square waffle maker and grease with cooking spray.
2. Pour Chaffle batter into the skillet and cook for about 3 minutes.
3. Meanwhile, heat oil in a pan over medium heat.
4. Once the oil is hot, add chicken thigh and garlic then, cook for about 5 minutes. Flip and cook for another 3–4 minutes.
5. Season with salt and pepper and give them a good mix.
6. Transfer cooked thigh to plate.
7. Fry the egg in the same pan for about 1–2 minutes according to your choice.
8. Once chaffles are cooked, serve with a fried egg and chicken thigh.
9. Enjoy!

Nutrition:

- **Calories**: 292
- **Protein**: 31 g
- **Fat**: 66 g
- **Carbohydrates**: 2 g

216. CHAFFLE EGG SANDWICH

Preparation Time: 10 minutes

Cooking Time: 10 minutes

Servings: 2

Ingredients:

- 2 keto chaffle
- 2 slice cheddar cheese
- 1 simple egg omelet

Directions:

1. Prepare your oven at 400°F.
2. Arrange egg omelet and cheese slice between chaffles.
3. Bake in the preheated oven for about 4–5 minutes until cheese is melted.
4. Once the cheese is melted, remove it from the oven.
5. Serve and enjoy!

Nutrition:

- **Calories**: 144
- **Protein**: 29 g
- **Fat**: 16 g
- **Carbohydrates**: 3 g

Preparation Time: 10 minutes

Cooking Time: 10 minutes

Servings: 2

Ingredients:

- 1 large egg
- 1/8 cup almond flour
- ½ tsp. garlic powder
- 3/4 tsp. baking powder
- ½ cup shredded cheese

Sandwich Filling:

- 2 slices deli ham
- 2 slices tomatoes
- 1 slice cheddar cheese

Directions:

1. Grease your square waffle maker and preheat it on medium heat.
2. Mix together chaffle ingredients in a mixing bowl until well combined.
3. Pour batter into a square waffle and make two chaffles.
4. Once chaffles are cooked, remove them from the maker.
5. For a sandwich, arrange deli ham, tomato slice, and cheddar cheese between two chaffles.
6. Cut sandwich from the center.
7. Serve and enjoy!

Nutrition:

- **Calories:** 159
- **Protein:** 29 g
- **Fat:** 66 g
- **Carbohydrates:** 4 g

Preparation Time: 10 minutes

Cooking Time: 10 minutes

Servings: 1

Ingredients:

- 2 square keto chaffle
- 2 slice cheddar cheese
- 2 lettuce leaves

Directions:

1. Prepare your oven at 400°F.
2. Arrange lettuce leave and cheese slice between chaffles.
3. Bake in the preheated oven for about 4–5 minutes until cheese is melted.
4. Once the cheese is melted, remove it from the oven.
5. Serve and enjoy!

Nutrition:

- **Calories**: 149
- **Protein**: 28 g
- **Fat**: 69 g
- **Carbohydrates**: 3 g

219. CHICKEN ZINGER CHAFFLE

Preparation Time: 10 minutes

Cooking Time: 15 minutes

Servings: 2

Ingredients:

- 1 chicken breast, cut into 2 pieces
- ½ cup coconut flour
- ¼ cup finely grated Parmesan
- 1 tsp. paprika
- ½ tsp. garlic powder
- ½ tsp. onion powder
- 1 tsp. salt & pepper
- 1 egg beaten
- Avocado oil for frying
- Lettuce leaves
- BBQ sauce

Chaffle Ingredients:

- 4 oz. cheese
- 2 whole eggs
- 2 oz. almond flour
- ¼ cup almond flour
- 1 tsp. baking powder

Directions:

1. Mix together chaffle ingredients in a bowl.
2. Pour the chaffle batter into preheated greased square chaffle maker.
3. Cook chaffles for about 2-minutes until cooked through.
4. Make square chaffles from this batter.
5. Meanwhile, mix together coconut flour, parmesan, paprika, garlic powder, onion powder, salt, and pepper in a bowl.
6. Dip chicken first in coconut flour mixture then in beaten egg.

7. Heat avocado oil in a skillet and cook chicken from both sides. until lightly brown and cooked.

8. Set chicken zinger between two chaffles with lettuce and BBQ sauce.

9. Enjoy!

Nutrition:

- **Calories**: 219
- **Protein**: 30 g
- **Fat**: 60 g
- **Carbohydrates**: 9 g

Preparation Time: 10 minutes

Cooking Time: 5 minutes

Servings: 2

Ingredients:

- ½ cup boil shredded chicken
- ¼ cup cheddar cheese
- 1/8 cup parmesan cheese
- 1 egg
- 1 tsp. Italian seasoning
- 1/8 tsp. garlic powder
- 1 tsp. cream cheese

Directions:

1. Preheat the Belgian waffle maker.
2. Mix together in chaffle ingredients in a bowl and mix together.
3. Sprinkle 1 tbsp. of cheese in a waffle maker and pour in chaffle batter.
4. Pour 1 tbsp. of cheese over batter and close the lid.
5. Cook chaffles for about 4 to minute.
6. Serve with a chicken zinger and enjoy the double chicken flavor.

Nutrition:

- **Calories:** 129
- **Protein:** 30 g
- **Fat:** 65 g
- **Carbohydrates:** 5 g

Preparation Time: 10 minutes

Cooking Time: 10 minutes

Servings: 2

Ingredients:

- 1 large egg
- 1 tbsp. almond flour
- 1 tbsp. full-fat Greek yogurt
- 1/8 tsp. baking powder
- ¼ cup shredded Swiss cheese

Topping:

- 4oz. grill prawns
- 4 oz. steamed cauliflower mash
- ½ zucchini sliced
- 3 lettuce leaves
- 1 tomato, sliced
- 1 tbsp. flax seeds

Directions:

1. Make 3 chaffles with the given chaffles ingredients.
2. For serving, arrange lettuce leaves on each chaffle.
3. Top with zucchini slice, grill prawns, cauliflower mash, and a tomato slice.
4. Drizzle flax seeds on top.
5. Serve and enjoy!

Nutrition:

- **Calories:** 75
- **Protein:** 45 g
- **Fat:** 47 g
- **Carbohydrates:** 8 g

Preparation Time: 10 minutes

Cooking Time: 15 minutes

Servings: 2

Ingredients:

- 1 egg
- ½ cup cheddar cheese, shredded
- 1 tbsp. parmesan cheese
- 3/4 tsp. coconut flour
- ¼ tsp. baking powder
- 1/8 tsp. Italian seasoning
- Pinch salt
- ¼ tsp. garlic powder

For Topping

- 1 bacon sliced, cooked, and chopped
- ½ cup mozzarella cheese, shredded
- ¼ tsp. parsley, chopped

Directions:

1. Preheat oven to 400°F.
2. Switch on your waffle maker and grease with cooking spray.
3. Mix together chaffle ingredients in a mixing bowl until combined.
4. Spoon half of the batter in the center of the waffle maker and close the lid. Cook the chaffles for about 3-minutes until cooked.
5. Carefully remove chaffles from the maker.
6. Arrange chaffles in a greased baking tray.
7. Top with mozzarella cheese, chopped bacon, and parsley.
8. And bake in the oven for 4–5 minutes.
9. Once the cheese is melted, remove it from the oven.
10. Serve and enjoy!

Nutrition:

- **Calories:** 222
- **Protein:** 28 g
- **Fat:** 69 g
- **Carbohydrates:** 3 g

Preparation Time: 10 minutes

Cooking Time: 10 minutes

Servings: 1

Ingredients:

- 1 beefsteak rib eye
- 1 tsp. salt
- 1 tsp. pepper
- 1 tbsp. lime juice
- 1 tsp. garlic

Directions:

1. Prepare your grill for direct heat.
2. Mix together all spices and rub over beefsteak evenly.
3. Place the beef on the grill rack over medium heat.
4. Cover and cook steak for about 6 to 8 minutes. Flip and cook for another 5 minutes, until cooked through.
5. Serve with simple keto chaffle, and enjoy!

Nutrition:

- **Calories:** 274
- **Protein:** 51 g
- **Fat:** 45 g
- **Carbohydrates:** 4 g

Preparation Time: 10 minutes

Cooking Time: 15 minutes

Servings: 2

Ingredients:

- ½ cup cauliflower
- ¼ tsp. garlic powder
- ¼ tsp. black pepper
- ¼ tsp. salt
- ½ cup shredded cheddar cheese
- 1 egg

For Topping:

- 1 lettuce leave
- 1 tomato sliced
- 4 oz. cauliflower steamed, mashed
- 1 tsp. sesame seeds

Directions:

1. Add all chaffle ingredients into a blender and mix well.
2. Sprinkle 1/8 shredded cheese on the waffle maker and pour cauliflower mixture in a preheated waffle maker and sprinkle the rest of the cheese over it.
3. Cook chaffles for about 4–5 minutes, until cooked
4. For serving, lay lettuce leaves over chaffle top with steamed cauliflower and tomato.
5. Drizzle sesame seeds on top.
6. Enjoy!

Nutrition:

- **Calories**: 128
- **Protein**: 25 g
- **Fat**: 65 g
- **Carbohydrates**: 10 g

Preparation Time: 10 minutes

Cooking Time: 15 minutes

Servings: 2

Ingredients:

- 4 eggs
- 2 cups grated mozzarella cheese
- Salt and pepper to taste
- Pinch nutmeg
- 2 tbsp. sour cream
- 6 tbsp. almond flour
- 2 tsp. baking powder
- Pork chops
- 2 tbsp. olive oil
- 1 pound pork chops
- Salt and pepper to taste
- 1 tsp. freshly chopped rosemary

Other:

- 2 tbsp. cooking spray to brush the waffle maker
- 2 tbsp. freshly chopped basil for decoration

Directions:

1. Preheat the waffle maker.
2. Add the eggs, mozzarella cheese, salt and pepper, nutmeg, sour cream, almond flour, and baking powder to a bowl.
3. Mix until combined.
4. Brush the heated waffle maker with cooking spray and add a few tbsp. of the batter.
5. Close the lid and cook for about 7 minutes, depending on your waffle maker.
6. Meanwhile, heat the butter in a nonstick grill pan and season the pork chops with salt and pepper and freshly chopped rosemary.
7. Cook the pork chops for about 4–5 minutes on each side.

8. Serve each chaffle with a pork chop and sprinkle some freshly chopped basil on top.

Nutrition:

- **Calories**: 666
- **Fat**: 55.2 g
- **Carbohydrates**: 4.8 g
- **Protein**: 37.5 g

Preparation Time: 10 minutes

Cooking Time: 10 minutes

Servings: 2

Ingredients:

Batter:

- ½ pound ground beef
- 4 eggs
- 4 ounces cream cheese
- 1 cup grated mozzarella cheese
- Salt and pepper to taste
- 1 clove garlic, minced
- ½ tsp. freshly chopped rosemary

Other:

- 2 tbsp. butter to brush the waffle maker
- ¼ cup sour cream
- 2 tbsp. freshly chopped parsley for garnish

Directions:

1. Preheat the waffle maker.
2. Add the ground beef, eggs, cream cheese, grated mozzarella cheese, salt and pepper, minced garlic, and freshly chopped rosemary to a bowl.
3. Brush the heated waffle maker with butter and add a few tbsp. of the batter.
4. Close the lid and cook for about 8–10 minutes, depending on your waffle maker.
5. Serve each chaffle with a tbsp. of sour cream and freshly chopped parsley on top.
6. Serve and enjoy.

Nutrition:

- **Calories:** 368
- **Fat:** 24 g
- **Carbohydrates:** 2.1 g
- **Protein:** 27.4 g

Preparation Time: 10 minutes

Cooking Time: 15 minutes

Servings: 2

Ingredients:

Batter:

- 4 eggs
- ¼ cup cream cheese
- 1 cup grated mozzarella cheese
- Salt and pepper to taste
- ¼ cup almond flour
- 1 tsp. freshly chopped dill

Beef:

- 1 pound beef loin
- Salt and pepper to taste
- 1 tbsp. balsamic vinegar
- 2 tbsp. olive oil
- 1 tsp. freshly chopped rosemary

Other:

- 2 tbsp. cooking spray to brush the waffle maker
- 4 tomato slices for serving

Directions:

1. Preheat the waffle maker.
2. Add the eggs, cream cheese, grated mozzarella cheese, salt and pepper, almond flour, and freshly chopped dill to a bowl.
3. Mix until combined and batter forms.
4. Brush the heated waffle maker with cooking spray and add a few tbsp. of the batter.
5. Close the lid and cook for about 8–10 minutes, depending on your waffle maker.

6. Meanwhile, heat the olive oil in a nonstick frying pan and season the beef loin with salt and pepper and freshly chopped rosemary.

7. Cook the beef on each side for about 5 minutes and drizzle with some balsamic vinegar.

8. Serve each chaffle with a slice of tomato and cooked beef loin slices.

Nutrition:

- **Calories:** 402
- **Fat:** 35.8 g
- **Carbohydrates:** 3.3 g
- **Protein:** 40.3 g

Preparation Time: 10 minutes

Cooking Time: 15 minutes

Servings: 2

Ingredients:

- ½ pound ground pork
- 3 eggs
- ½ cup grated mozzarella cheese
- Salt and pepper to taste
- 1 clove garlic, minced
- 1 tsp. dried oregano

Other:

- 2 tbsp. butter to brush the waffle maker
- 2 tbsp. freshly chopped parsley for garnish

Directions:

1. Preheat the waffle maker.
2. Add the ground pork, eggs, mozzarella cheese, salt and pepper, minced garlic, and dried oregano to a bowl.
3. Mix until combined.
4. Brush the heated waffle maker with butter and add a few tbsp. of the batter.
5. Close the lid and cook for about 7–8 minutes, depending on your waffle maker.
6. Serve with freshly chopped parsley.

Nutrition:

- **Calories**: 192
- **Fat**: 11 g
- **Carbohydrates**: 1 g
- **Protein**: 20.2 g

Preparation Time: 10 minutes

Cooking Time: 10 minutes

Servings: 1

Ingredients:

- 1 egg
- 1 oz. cream cheese, softened
- 1 cup cheddar cheese, shredded

For the Toppings:

- 2 tbsp. bacon bits
- ½ tbsp. jalapenos

Directions:

1. Turn on the waffle maker. Preheat for up to 5 minutes.
2. Mix the chaffle ingredients.
3. Pour the batter onto the waffle maker.
4. Cook the batter for 3–4 minutes until it's brown and crispy.
5. Remove the chaffle and repeat steps until all remaining batter has been used up.
6. Sprinkle bacon bits and a few jalapeno slices as toppings.

Nutrition:

- **Calories**: 231
- **Carbohydrates**: 2 g
- **Fat**: 18 g
- **Protein**: 13 g

Preparation Time: 15 minutes

Cooking Time: 10 minutes

Servings: 1

Ingredients:

- 1 egg, separated
- 1 egg yolk
- ½ cup mozzarella cheese Shredded
- ½ tsp. spiced rum
- 1 tsp. vanilla extract
- ¼ tsp. nutmeg, dried
- A dash cinnamon
- 1 tsp. coconut flour

For the Icing:

- 2 tbsp. cream cheese
- 1 tbsp. powdered sweetener
- 2 tsp. rum or rum extract

Directions:

1. Preheat the mini waffle maker.
2. Mix egg yolk in a small bowl until smooth.
3. Add in the sweetener and mix until the powder is completely dissolved.
4. Add the coconut flour, cinnamon, and nutmeg. Mix well.
5. In another bowl, mix rum, egg white, and vanilla. Whisk until well combined.
6. Throw in the yolk mixture with the egg white mixture. You should be able to form a thin batter.
7. Add the mozzarella cheese and combine it with the mixture.
8. Separate the batter into two batches. Put ½ of the batter into the waffle maker and let it cook for 6 minutes until it's solid.
9. Repeat until you've used up the remaining batter.
10. In a separate bowl, mix all the icing ingredients.
11. Top the cooked chaffles with the icing, or you can use this as a dip.

Nutrition:

- **Calories:** 266
- **Carbohydrates:** 2 g
- **Fat:** 23 g
- **Protein:** 13 g

Preparation Time: 15 minutes

Cooking Time: 10 minutes

Servings: 1

Ingredients:

- 1 egg
- ½ cup cheddar cheese shredded
- 1 tbsp. almond flour
- 1 tbsp. jalapenos
- 1 tbsp. olive oil

Directions:

1. Preheat the waffle maker.
2. While waiting for the waffle maker to heat up, mix jalapeno, egg, cheese, and almond flour in a small mixing bowl.
3. Lightly grease the waffle maker with olive oil.
4. In the center of the waffle maker, carefully pour the chaffle batter. Spread the mixture evenly toward the edges.
5. Close the waffle maker lid and wait for 3-4 minutes for the mixture to cook. For an even crispier texture, wait for another 1–2 minutes.
6. Remove the chaffle. Let it cool before serving.

Nutrition:

- **Calories**: 509
- **Carbohydrates**: 5 g
- **Fat**: 45 g
- **Protein**: 23 g

Chapter 9.
OTHER CHAFFLES RECIPES

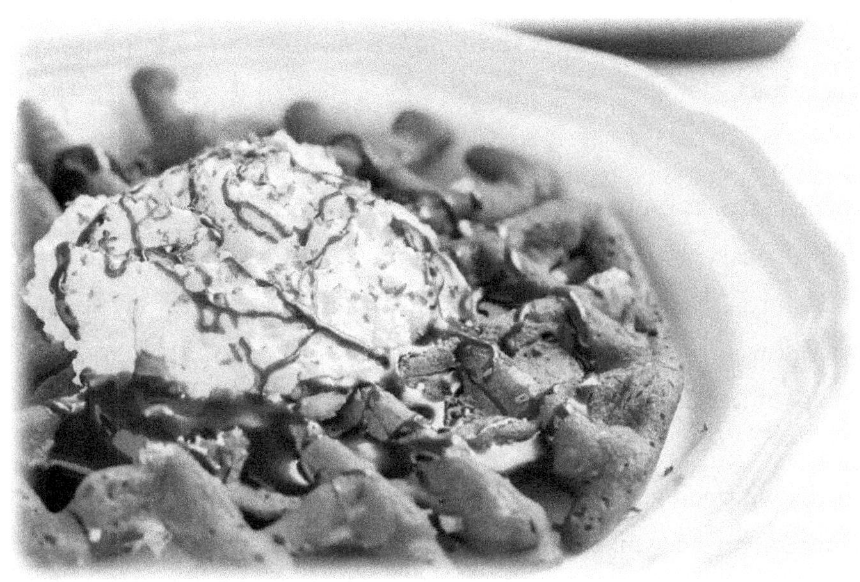

232. KETO BIRTHDAY CAKE CHAFFLE WITH SPRINKLES

Preparation Time: 10 minutes

Cooking Time: 7 minutes

Servings: 4

Ingredients:

For Chaffle Cake:

- 2 eggs
- ¼ almond flour
- 1 cup coconut powder
- 1 cup melted butter
- 2 tbsp. cream cheese
- 1 tsp. cake butter extract
- 1 tsp. vanilla extract

- 2 tsp. baking powder
- 2 tsp. confectionery sweetener or monk fruit
- ¼ tsp. xanthan powder whipped cream

Vanilla Frosting Ingredients:

- ½ cup heavy whipped cream
- 2 tbsp. sweetener or monk fruit
- ½ tsp. vanilla extract

Directions:

1. The mini waffle maker is preheated.
2. Add all the chaffle cake ingredients to a medium-sized blender and blend it to the top until it is smooth and creamy. Allow only a minute to sit with the batter. It may seem a little watery, but it's going to work well.
3. Add 2 to 3 tbsp. of batter to your waffle maker and cook until golden brown for about 2 to 3 minutes.
4. Start to frost the whipped vanilla cream in a separate bowl.
5. Add all the ingredients and mix with a hand mixer until the whipping cream forms thick and soft peaks.
6. Until frosting your cake, allow the keto birthday cake chaffles to cool completely. If you frost it too soon, the frosting will be melted.

Nutrition:

- **Calories**: 141
- **Fat**: 10.2 g
- **Protein**: 4.7 g
- **Carbohydrates**: 5 g

Preparation Time: 5 minutes

Cooking Time: 5 minutes

Servings: 3

Ingredients:

- 2 tbsp. cocoa
- 2 tbsp. monk fruit confectioner's
- 1 egg
- ¼ tsp. baking powder
- 1 tbsp. heavy whipped cream

Frosted Ingredients:

- 2 tbsp. monk fruit confectioners
- 2 tbsp. cream cheese softens, room temperature
- ¼ tsp. transparent vanilla

Directions:

1. Whip the egg.
2. Stir in the rest of the ingredients, then mix well until smooth and creamy.
3. Pour half of the batter into a mini waffle maker and cook until fully cooked for 2 ½ to 3 minutes.
4. Add the sweetener, cream cheese, and vanilla in a separate small bowl. Mix the frosting until all is well embedded.
5. Layout the frosting on the cake after it has cooled down to room temperature.

Nutrition:

- **Calories:** 120
- **Fat:** 10.5 g
- **Protein:** 4.1 g
- **Carbohydrates:** 8 g

Preparation Time: 5 minutes

Cooking Time: 5 minutes

Servings: 6

Ingredients:

- ½ cup chopped carrot
- 1 egg
- 2 tbsp. butter melted
- 2 tbsp. heavy whipped cream
- 3/4 cup almond flour
- 1 walnut chopped
- 2 tsp. powder sweetener
- 2 tsp. cinnamon
- 1 tsp. pumpkin spice
- 1 tsp. baking powder
- Cream cheese frosting
- 4 oz. cream cheese softened
- ¼ cup powdered sweetener
- 1 tsp. vanilla essence
- 1–2 tsp. heavy whipped cream according to your preferred consistency

Directions:

1. Mix dry ingredients such as almond flour, cinnamon, pumpkin spices, baking powder, powdered sweeteners, and walnut pieces.
2. Add the grated carrots, eggs, melted butter, and cream.
3. Add 3 tablespoons of batter to a preheated mini waffle maker. Cook for 2-½-3 minutes.
4. Mix the frosted ingredients with a hand mixer with a whisk until well mixed
5. Stack waffles and add a frost between each layer!

Nutrition:

- **Calories**: 120
- **Fat**: 12 g
- **Protein**: 5 g
- **Carbohydrates**: 6 g

Preparation Time: 5 minutes

Cooking Time: 12 minutes

Servings: 3

Ingredients:

- 1 egg
- ½ cup mozzarella cheese
- ½ tsp. vanilla
- ½ tsp. cinnamon
- 1 tbsp. monk fruit confectioner's blend

Directions:

1. Put the eggs in a small bowl.
2. Add the remaining ingredients.
3. Spray to the waffle maker with a non-stick cooking spray.
4. Make two chaffles.
5. Separate the mixture.
6. Cook half of the mixture for about 4 minutes or until golden.
7. Notes added glaze: 1 tbsp. of cream cheese melted in a microwave for 15 seconds, and 1 tbsp. of monk fruit confectioners' mix. Mix it and spread it over the moist fabric.
8. Additional frosting: 1 tbsp. cream cheese (high temp), 1 tbsp. room temp butter (low temp) and 1 tbsp. monk fruit confectioners' mix. Mix all the ingredients together and spread to the top of the cloth.
9. Top with optional frosting, glaze, nuts, sugar-free syrup, whipped cream, or simply dust with monk fruit sweets.

Nutrition:

- **Calories:** 106
- **Fat:** 6.6 g
- **Protein:** 8.2 g
- **Carbohydrates:** 4 g

Preparation Time: 5 minutes

Cooking Time: 5 minutes

Servings: 2

Ingredients:

- 1 large egg yolk
- ½ cup fresh cream
- 3 tbsp. powder sweetener
- ¼–½ tsp. xanthan gum
- ½ tsp. banana extract

Banana Chaffle Ingredients:

- 1 oz. softened cream cheese
- ¼ cup mozzarella cheese shredded
- 1 egg
- 1 tsp. banana extract
- 2 t sweetener
- 1 tsp. baking powder
- 4 t almond flour

Directions:

1. Mix heavy cream, powdered sweetener, and egg yolk in a small pot. Whisk constantly until the sweetener has dissolved and the mixture is thick.
2. Cook for 1 minute. Add xanthan gum and whisk.
3. Remove from heat, add a pinch of salt and banana extract, and stir well.
4. Transfer to a glass dish and cover the pudding with plastic wrap. Refrigerate.
5. Mix all ingredients together. Cook in a preheated mini waffle maker.

Nutrition:

- **Calories:** 130
- **Fat:** 13 g
- **Protein:** 4 g
- **Carbohydrates:** 5 g

Preparation Time: 5 minutes

Cooking Time: 5 minutes

Servings: 2

Ingredients:

For Peanut Butter Chaffle:

- 2 tbsp. sugar-free peanut butter powder
- 2 tbsp. monk fruit confectioner's
- 1 egg
- ¼ tsp. baking powder
- 1 tbsp. heavy whipped cream
- ¼ tsp. peanut butter extract

Peanut Butter Frosting Ingredients:

- 2 tbsp. monk fruit confectioners
- 1 tbsp. butter softens, room temperature
- 1 tbsp. unsweetened natural peanut butter or peanut butter powder
- 2 tbsp. cream cheese softens, room temperature
- ¼ tsp. vanilla

Directions:

1. Serve the eggs.
2. Stir in the remaining ingredients, then mix well until smooth and creamy.
3. If you don't have peanut butter extract, you can skip it. It adds absolutely wonderful, more powerful peanut butter flavor and is worth investing in this extract.
4. Pour half of the butter into a mini waffle maker and cook for 2–3 minutes until it is completely cooked.
5. In another small bowl, add sweetener, cream cheese, sugar-free natural peanut butter, and vanilla. Mix frosting until everything is well incorporated.
6. When the waffle cake has completely cooled to room temperature, spread the frosting.
7. Or you can even pipe the frost!

8. Or you can warm up the frosting and pour ½ tsp. of water to make the peanut butter and drizzle over the peanut butter chaffle! I like it anyway!

Nutrition:

- **Calories**: 92
- **Fat**: 7 g
- **Protein**: 5.5 g
- **Carbohydrates**: 6 g

Preparation Time: 5 minutes

Cooking Time: 3 minutes

Servings: 1

Ingredients:

For Sweet Chaffle:

- 4 oz. cream cheese softens, room temperature
- 4 eggs
- 1 tbsp. butter
- 1 tsp. vanilla essence
- ½ tsp. cinnamon
- 1 tbsp. monk fruit sweetener or favorite keto-approved sweetener
- 4 tbsp. coconut powder
- 1 tbsp. almond flour
- 1 ½ cup baking powder
- 1 tbsp. coconut
- 1 walnut chopped

Italian Cream Frosting:

- 2 oz. cream cheese softens, room temperature
- 2 cups of butter room temp
- 2 tbsp. monk fruit sweetener or favorite keto-approved sweetener
- ½ tsp. vanilla

Directions:

1. Using a medium blender, stir in cream cheese, eggs, melted butter, vanilla, sweeteners, coconut flour, almond flour, and baking powder.
2. Optional: add shredded coconut and walnut to the mixture or save for matting. Both methods are great!
3. Incorporate the ingredients high until smooth and creamy.
4. Heat up mini waffle maker.
5. Pour in ingredients to the preheated waffle maker.

6. Cook for 3 minutes until the waffle is complete.

7. Take out the chaffle and let it cool.

8. Mix all the ingredients together and start frosting. Stir until smooth.

9. Once cooled, frost the cake.

Nutrition:

- **Calories**: 127
- **Fat**: 9.7 g
- **Protein**: 5.3 g
- **Carbohydrates**: 11 g

Preparation Time: 10 minutes

Cooking Time: 5 minutes

Servings: 4

Ingredients:

For Chaffle Cake:

- 2 eggs
- ¼ cup almond flour
- Coconut flower 1 tsp.
- 2 tbsp. melted butter
- 2 tbsp. cream cheese
- 20 drops Boston cream extract
- ½ tsp. vanilla essence
- ½ tsp. baking powder
- 2 tbsp. sweetener or monk fruit
- ¼ tsp. xanthan powder

Custard Ingredients:

- ½ cup fresh cream
- ½ tsp. vanilla essence
- ½ tbsp. swerve confectioner's sweetener
- 2 yolks
- 1/8 tsp. xanthan gum

For Ganache:

- 2 tbsp. heavy whipped cream
- 2 tbsp. unsweetened baking chocolate bar chopped
- 1 tbsp. swerve confectioners' sweetener

Directions:

1. Preheat the mini waffle iron to render the cake chops first.
2. Using a mixer, blend all the ingredients of the cake and blend until smooth. It's only supposed to take a few minutes.

3. Warm-up heavy whipping cream to a boil on the stovetop. While it's dry, whisk the egg yolks together in a small separate dish.

4. Once the cream is boiling, add half of it to the egg yolks. Make sure you're whisking it together while you're slowly pouring it into the mixture.

5. Beat egg and milk mixture to the rest of the cream in the stovetop pan and stir vigorously for 4 minutes.

6. Pull the custard off the heat and whisk in your vanilla and xanthan gum. Then set aside to cool and thicken.

7. Place the ganache ingredients in a small bowl. Microwave for about 20 seconds, stir. Repeat, if necessary. Careful not to overheat and roast the ganache. Just do it 20 seconds at a time until it's completely melted.

8. Assemble and enjoy your Boston cream pie chaffle cake!

Nutrition:

- **Calories**: 120
- **Fat**: 10.5 g
- **Protein**: 3 g
- **Carbohydrates**: 5 g

Preparation Time: 10 minutes

Cooking Time: 5 minutes

Servings: 4

Ingredients:

For Chaffle Cake:

- 2 eggs
- ¼ cup almond flour
- Coconut flower 1 tsp.
- 2 tbsp. melted butter
- 2 tbsp. cream cheese
- 1 tsp. cake batter extract
- ½ tsp. vanilla essence
- ½ tsp. baking powder
- 2 tbsp. sweetener or monk fruit
- ¼ tsp. xanthan powder

Whipped Cream Vanilla Frosting:

- ½ cup fresh cream
- 2 tbsp. sweets sweetener or monk fruit
- ½ tsp. vanilla essence

Directions:

1. Preheat mini waffle maker.
2. In a medium-sized blender, add all the chaffle cake ingredients and blend high until smooth and creamy. Let the dough sit for only one minute. It may look a bit watery, but it works.
3. Add 2–3 tablespoons of dough to the waffle maker and cook for about 2–3 minutes until golden.
4. In another bowl, start making the whipped cream vanilla frosting.
5. Add all ingredients and mix with a hand mixer until whipped cream thickens and soft peaks form.

6. Let the keto birthday cake chaffle cool completely before frosting the cake. If the frost is too early, the frost will melt.

Nutrition:

- **Calories**: 141
- **Fat**: 10.2 g
- **Protein**: 4.7 g
- **Carbohydrates**: 6 g

Preparation Time: 2 minutes

Cooking Time: 4 minutes

Servings: 2

Ingredients:

- 1 egg
- 1 tbsp. heavy whipped cream
- 1 tsp. coconut flour
- 2 tbsp. Lecanto golden sweetener (use off wine)
- ½ tsp. cake batter extract
- ¼ tsp. baking powder

Directions:

1. Preheat the maker of mini waffles.
2. Combine all the ingredients of the chaffle in a small bowl.
3. Pour half of the mixture of the chaffle into the waffle iron center. Allow 3–5 minutes to cook. If the chaffle rises, lift the lid slightly for a couple of seconds until it begins to go back down and restore the lid as it finishes.
4. Carefully remove the second chaffle and repeat it. Let the chaffles sit for a couple of minutes to crisp up.
5. Add your desired and enjoyed the amount of whipped cream and strawberries!
6. Notes: recipe is perfect in a standard waffle maker for either two mini chaffles or one chaffle.
7. The calculated macros on the bottom are before the amount of strawberries and whipped cream you want.

Nutrition:

- **Calories:** 268
- **Fat:** 11.8 g
- **Protein:** 10 g
- **Carbohydrates:** 8 g

242. LEMON CAKE CHAFFLE

Preparation Time: 10 minutes

Cooking Time: 28 minutes

Servings: 4

Ingredients:

For the chaffles:

- 2 eggs, beaten
- ½ cup finely grated swiss cheese
- 2 oz. cream cheese, softened
- ½ tsp. lemon extract
- 20 drops cake batter extract

For the Frosting:

- ½ cup heavy cream
- 1 tbsp. sugar-free maple syrup
- ¼ tsp. lemon extract

Directions:

For the Chaffles:

1. Preheat the waffle iron.
2. Incorporate all the ingredients for the chaffles.
3. Open the iron and add a quarter of the mixture. Close and cook until crispy, 7 minutes.
4. Transfer the chaffle to a plate and make 3 more chaffles with the remaining batter.

For the Frosting:

1. Using a hand mixer, a medium bowl, beat the heavy cream, maple syrup, and lemon extract until fluffy.
2. Assemble the chaffles with the frosting to make the cake.
3. Slice and serve.

Nutrition:

- **Calories:** 176
- **Fat:** 15.18 g
- **Protein:** 7.63 g
- **Carbohydrates:** 5 g

Preparation Time: 15 minutes

Cooking Time: 28 minutes

Servings: 4

Ingredients:

For the Chaffles:

- 2 eggs, beaten
- ½ cup finely grated parmesan cheese
- 2 oz. cream cheese, softened
- 2 drops red food coloring
- 1 tsp. vanilla extract

For the Frosting:

- 3 tbsp. cream cheese, softened
- 1 tbsp. sugar-free maple syrup
- ¼ tsp. vanilla extract

Directions:

For the Chaffles:

1. Preheat the waffle iron.
2. Incorporate all the ingredients for the chaffles.
3. Open the iron and add a quarter of the mixture. Close and cook until crispy, 7 minutes.
4. Transfer the chaffle to a plate and make 3 more chaffles with the remaining batter.

For the Frosting:

1. In a medium bowl, using a hand mixer, whisk the cream cheese, maple syrup, and vanilla extract until smooth.
2. Assemble the chaffles with the frosting to make the cake.
3. Slice and serve.

Nutrition:

- **Calories:** 147
- **Fat:** 9.86 g
- **Protein:** 8.57 g
- **Carbohydrates:** 11 g

Preparation Time: 20 minutes

Cooking Time: 28 minutes

Servings: 4

Ingredients:

For the Chaffles:

- 1 egg, beaten
- 1/3 cup finely grated mozzarella cheese
- 1 tbsp. almond flour
- 2 tbsp. almond butter
- 1 tbsp. swerve confectioner's sugar
- ½ tsp. vanilla extract

For the Chocolate Butter Frosting:

- 1½ cups butter, room temperature
- 1 cup unsweetened cocoa powder
- ½ cup almond milk
- 5 cups swerve confectioner's sugar
- 2 tsp. vanilla extract

Directions:

For the Chaffles:

1. Preheat the waffle iron.
2. In a medium bowl, mix the egg, mozzarella cheese, almond flour, almond butter, swerve confectioner's sugar, and vanilla extract.
3. Open the iron and add a quarter of the mixture. Close and cook until crispy, 7 minutes.
4. Transfer the chaffle to a plate and make 3 more chaffles with the remaining batter.

For the Frosting:

1. Whisk butter and cocoa powder until smooth.
2. Gradually, whisk in the almond milk and swerve confectioner's sugar until smooth.
3. Add the vanilla extract and mix well.

4. Assemble the chaffles with the frosting to make the cake.

5. Slice and serve.

Nutrition:

- **Calories**: 838
- **Fat**: 8.35 g
- **Protein**: 13.59 g
- **Carbohydrates**: 15 g

Preparation Time: 5 minutes

Cooking Time: 15 minutes

Servings: 4

Ingredients:

- 4 large eggs
- 1 cup shredded cheese
- 2 tbsps. coconut cream
- 2 tbsps. Coconut flour.
- 1 tsp. stevia

Topping:

- 1 cup heavy cream
- 8 oz. raspberries
- 4 oz. blueberries
- 2 oz. cherries

Directions:

1. Make 4 thin round chaffles with the chaffle ingredients. Once chaffles are cooked, set in layers on a plate.
2. Spread heavy cream in each layer.
3. Top with raspberries, then blueberries and cherries.
4. Serve and enjoy!

Nutrition:

- **Calories:** 318
- **Fat:** 26.05 g
- **Protein:** 15.7 g
- **Carbohydrates:** 13 g

Preparation Time: 5 minutes

Cooking Time: 15 minutes

Servings: 5

Ingredients:

- 4 oz. almond flour
- 2 cup cheddar cheese
- 5 eggs
- 1 tsp. stevia
- 2 tsp. baking powder
- 2 tsp. vanilla extract
- ¼ cup almond butter, melted
- 3 tbsps. almond milk
- 1 cup cranberries
- 1 cup coconut cream

Directions:

1. Beat eggs in a bowl, incorporate almond flour, stevia, and baking powder.
2. Pour in melted butter slowly into the flour mixture until smooth consistency.
3. Add the cheese, almond milk, cranberries, and vanilla to the flour and butter mixture; be sure to mix well.
4. Preheat the waffles maker according to manufacturer instruction and grease it with avocado oil.
5. Fill in the batter into the waffle maker, then cook until golden brown.
6. Make 5 chaffles.
7. Stag chaffles in a plate. Spread the cream all around.
8. Cut in slice and serve.

Nutrition:

- **Calories:** 243
- **Fat:** 42.4 g
- **Protein:** 7.87 g
- **Carbohydrates:** 5 g

Preparation Time: 5 minutes

Cooking Time: 5 minutes

Servings: 8

Ingredients:

- 8 keto chocolate square chaffles
- 2 cups peanut butter
- 16 oz. raspberries

Directions:

1. Assemble chaffles in layers.
2. Spread peanut butter in each layer.
3. Top with raspberries.
4. Enjoy cake on Christmas morning with keto coffee!

Nutrition:

- **Calories:** 243
- **Fat:** 42 g
- **Protein:** 7.87 g
- **Carbohydrates:** 4 g

Preparation Time: 20 minutes

Cooking Time: 20 minutes

Servings: 4

Ingredients:

- 4 oz. cream cheese, at room temp
- 4 eggs
- 1 tbsp. melted butter
- 1 tsp. vanilla extract
- ½ tsp. cinnamon
- 1 tbsp. monk fruit sweetener
- 4 tbsp. coconut flour
- 1 tbsp. almond flour
- 1½ tsp. baking powder
- 1 tbsp. coconut, shredded, and unsweetened
- 1 tbsp. walnuts, chopped

For the Italian Cream Frosting:

- 2 oz. cream cheese, at room temp
- 2 tbsp. butter room temp
- 2 tbsp. monk fruit sweetener
- ½ tsp. vanilla

Directions:

1. Combine cream cheese, eggs, melted butter, vanilla, sweetener, flours, and baking powder in a blender.
2. Add walnuts and coconut to the mixture.
3. Blend to get a creamy mixture.
4. Turn on the waffle maker to heat and oil it with cooking spray.
5. Add enough batter to fill the waffle maker. Cook for 2–3 minutes until the chaffles are done.
6. Remove and let them cool.
7. Mix all frosting ingredients in another bowl. Stir until smooth and creamy.

8. Frost the chaffles once they have cooled.

9. Top with cream and more nuts.

Nutrition:

- **Calories**: 168
- **Fat**: 2 g
- **Protein**: 5 g
- **Carbohydrates**: 8 g

Preparation Time: 10 minutes

Cooking Time: 30 minutes

Servings: 4

Ingredients:

- 2 eggs
- 2 oz. cream cheese, softened
- 1 tbsp. coconut flour
- 2 tsp. heavy cream
- 2 tsp. lemon juice
- ½ tsp. vanilla extract
- ¼ tsp. stevia powder
- ¼ tsp. baking soda
- 8 oz. cream cheese, softened
- 2 oz. unsalted butter, softened
- 1 tbsp. stevia powder
- 1 tbsp. lemon zest
- 1 tsp. lemon juice
- ½ tsp. vanilla extract

Directions:

1. Preheat the mini waffle maker.
2. Combine all the chaffle ingredients using a blender.
3. Onto the preheated waffle maker, pour ¼ of the batter.
4. Close the lid. Let the batter cook for 4–5 minutes. Remove the cooked chaffle using a pair of silicone tongs.
5. Repeat the steps to use up the remaining batter.
6. Let the chaffles cool completely.
7. Make the lemon frosting by combining the ingredients in a bowl.
8. Assemble by cutting two of the chaffles in half.
9. Use cling wrap to line a small bowl.
10. Place a whole chaffle in the bowl, carefully molding it to the shape of the bowl.

11. Line each side with the four chaffle halves.

12. Add half the amount of lemon frosting.

13. Cover the frosting with the last whole chaffle.

14. Cover the bowl with cling wrap. Put in the fridge for 30 minutes. You don't need to chill the remaining lemon frosting.

15. Invert the chaffle dome onto a plate.

16. Spread the remaining lemon frosting over it. Add decorations if desired.

17. Chill the cake for another 30 minutes. Serve.

Nutrition:

- **Calories:** 405
- **Fat:** 38 g
- **Protein:** 9 g
- **Carbohydrates:** 13 g

Preparation Time: 15 minutes

Cooking Time: 10 minutes

Servings: 1

Ingredients:

- 1 egg
- 2 tbsp. almond flour
- ½ tsp. coconut flour
- 1 tbsp. butter, melted
- 1 tbsp. cream cheese, softened
- ¼ tsp. vanilla extract
- ¼ tsp. baking powder
- 1 tbsp. confectioners' sweetener
- 1/8 tsp. xanthan gum
- 20 drops captain cereal flavoring
- Whipped cream

Directions:

1. Preheat the mini waffle maker.
2. Blend or mix all the chaffles ingredients until the consistency is creamy and smooth. Set aside for a few minutes so that the flour absorbs the liquid ingredients.
3. Scoop out 2–3 tablespoons of batter and put it into the waffle maker. Allow cooking for 2–3 minutes.
4. Top the cooked chaffles with freshly whipped cream.
5. Add syrup and drops of Captain Cereal flavoring for a great flavor.

Nutrition:

- **Calories:** 154
- **Fat:** 11.2 g
- **Protein:** 4.6 g
- **Carbohydrates:** 9 g

Preparation Time: 7 minutes

Cooking Time: 12 minutes

Servings: 4

Ingredients:

For Chaffle:

- 4 oz. cream cheese, softened
- 4 eggs
- 4 tbsp. coconut flour
- 1 tbsp. almond flour
- 1 ½ tsp. baking powder
- 1 tbsp. butter, softened
- 1 tsp. vanilla extract
- ½ tsp. cinnamon
- 1 tbsp. sweetener
- 1 tbsp. shredded coconut, colored and unsweetened
- 1 tbsp. walnuts, chopped

For Italian Cream Frosting:

- 2 oz. cream cheese, softened
- 2 tbsp. butter, room temperature
- 2 tbsp. sweetener
- ½ tsp. vanilla

Directions:

1. Add the almond flour, coconut flour, eggs, cream cheese, softened butter, vanilla, sweetener, and baking powder in a blender and blend until smooth.
2. Add the walnuts and shredded coconut to the mixture.
3. Blend the ingredients on the high setting until you have a creamy mixture.
4. Preheat your waffle maker and add ¼ of the ingredients.
5. Cook for 3 minutes and repeat the process until you have 4 chaffles.
6. Remove and set aside.

7. In the meantime, start making your frosting by mixing all the ingredients together.

8. Stir until you have a smooth and creamy mixture.

9. Cool, frost the cake, and enjoy.

Nutrition:

- **Calories**: 127
- **Fat**: 10 g
- **Protein**: 7 g
- **Carbohydrates**: 5 g

Preparation Time: 5 minutes

Cooking Time: 12 minutes

Servings: 3

Ingredients:

Strawberry Topping Ingredients:

- 3 fresh strawberries
- ½ tbsp. granulated swerve

Sweet Chaffle Ingredients:

- 1 tbsp. almond flour
- ½ cup mozzarella cheese
- 1 egg
- 1 tbsp. granulated swerve
- ¼ tsp. vanilla extract
- Keto Whipped Cream

Directions:

1. Warm-up your waffle maker.
2. Wash and cut your fresh strawberries. Put the strawberries in a small bowl and add ½ tbsp. granulated swerve. Incorporate the strawberries with the swerve and set them aside.
3. Mix almond flour, egg, mozzarella cheese, granulated swerve, and vanilla extract.
4. Fill in 1/3 of the batter into your mini waffle maker and cook for 3–4 minutes. Then cook another 1/3 of the batter and the rest of the batter to make 3 keto chaffles.
5. While cooking, create your keto whipped cream if you do not have any on hand.
6. Assemble your Strawberry Shortcake Chaffle by putting whipped cream and strawberries on top of your sweet chaffle. Then sprinkle the juice that will also be in the bowl with the strawberries on top.

Nutrition:

- **Calories:** 112
- **Protein:** 7 g
- **Fat:** 8 g
- **Carbohydrates:** 11 g

Preparation Time: 5 minutes

Cooking Time: 7 minutes

Servings: 6

Ingredients:

Cranberry Sauce:

- ½ cup cranberries fresh or frozen
- 2 tbsp. granulated erythritol
- ½ cup water
- ½ tsp. vanilla extract

Chaffles:

- 1 egg
- 1-ounce cream cheese at room temperature
- 1 tbsp. erythritol blends such as Swerve
- ½ tsp. vanilla extract
- 1 tsp. coconut flour
- ¼ tsp. baking powder

Frosting:

- 1-oz. cream cheese at room temp
- 1 tbsp. butter room temp
- 1 tbsp. Swerve
- 1/8 tsp. orange extract
- Grated orange zest (optional)

Directions:

1. For the cranberry swirl
2. Incorporate cranberries, water, and erythritol in a medium saucepan. Boil, then decrease the heat to a gentle simmer.
3. Simmer for 12 minutes, until the cranberries pop and the sauce thicken.
4. Pull away from heat, then stir in the vanilla extract.
5. Smash the berries with the back of a spoon until a chunky sauce forms.

For the Chaffles:

1.   Set up a mini-Dash waffle iron until thoroughly hot.
2.   Whisk all chaffle ingredients together until well combined.
3.   Ladle 2 tablespoons of batter into a waffle iron.
4.   Drizzle ½ of the cranberry sauce in little dollops over the batter of each chaffle.
5.   Cook for 3–5 minutes. Remove to a wire rack.
6.   Repeat for the second chaffle.

For the Frosting:

1.   Mix all ingredients, except orange zest, together until smooth and spread over each chaffle.
2.   Orange zest (optional).

Nutrition:

- **Calories**: 70
- **Protein**: 1.8 g
- **Fat**: 6 g
- **Carbohydrates**: 9 g

Preparation Time: 5 minutes

Cooking Time: 7 minutes

Servings: 5

Ingredients:

Apple Fritter Filling:

- 2 cups diced jicama
- ¼ cup plus 1 tbsp. Swerve sweetener blend
- 4 tbsp. butter
- 1 tsp. cinnamon
- 1/8 tsp. nutmeg
- Dash ground cloves
- ½ tsp. vanilla
- 20 drops Loran Oils apple flavoring

Chaffle:

- 2 eggs
- ½ cup mozzarella cheese
- 1 tbsp. almond flour
- 1 tsp. coconut flour
- ½ tsp. baking powder
- Glaze 1 tbsp. butter
- 2 tsp. heavy cream
- 3 tbsp. powdered sweetener such as Swerve Confectioners
- ¼ tsp. vanilla extract

Directions:

Keto Apple Fritter Chaffle Filling:

1. Skin the jicama and cut it into small dice.
2. Using a medium skillet over medium-low heat, melt the butter and add the diced jicama and sweetener.
3. Simmer slowly for 18 minutes, stirring often. Do not use high heat, so it doesn't overcook.

4. Once soft, remove from heat and stir in the spices and flavorings.

Keto Apple Fritter Chaffle:
1. Warm-up waffle iron until hot.
2. Whisk all ingredients except cheese. Stir the jicama mixture into the eggs.
3. Drizzle 1 tbsp. grated cheese on that waffle iron.
4. Ladle 2 heaping tbsp. of the egg/jicama mixture into the waffle iron and top with another tbsp. of cheese.
5. Cook for 6 minutes until nicely browned and crunchy.
6. Move it to a wire rack.

Keto Apple Fritter Chaffle Icing:

1. Melt butter in a small saucepan and add the Swerve and heavy cream.
2. Simmer at medium heat for 6 minutes.
3. Stir in vanilla.
4. Drizzle the hot icing over the chaffles. It will harden as it cools.

Nutrition:
- **Calories**: 186
- **Fat**: 14.3 g
- **Protein**: 7 g
- **Carbohydrates**: 11 g

Preparation Time: 5 minutes

Cooking Time: 7 minutes

Servings: 2

Ingredients:

Chaffle Batter:

- 1 large egg
- 2 oz. cream cheese softened
- ¼ tsp. pure vanilla extract
- 2 tbsp. Lecanto Confectioners Sweetener
- 1 oz. pork rinds crushed
- 1 tsp. baking powder

Marshmallow Frosting:

- ¼ c. Heavy Whipping Cream
- ¼ tsp. pure vanilla extract
- 1 tbsp. Lakanto Confectioners Sweetener
- ½ tsp. Xanthan gum

Directions:

1. Set up the mini waffle maker to preheat.
2. Incorporate egg, cream cheese, and vanilla.
3. Whisk well.
4. Stir in sweetener, crushed pork rinds, and baking powder.
5. Mix until well incorporated.
6. Stir in extra crushed pork rinds onto waffle maker (optional).
7. Pour in ¼ scoop of batter over, sprinkle a bit more pork rinds.
8. Cook 4 minutes, then remove and cool on a wire rack.
9. Do it for the remaining batter.

Marshmallow Frosting:

1. Whisk the HWC, vanilla, and confectioners until thick and fluffy.
2. Gradually drizzle over the xanthan gum and fold until well incorporated.

3. Layout frosting over the chaffles and cut as desired, then refrigerate until set.

Nutrition:

- **Calories**: 334
- **Protein**: 13 g
- **Fat**: 29 g
- **Carbohydrates**: 15 g

Preparation Time: 2 minutes

Cooking Time: 7 minutes

Servings: 2

Ingredients:

Chocolate Chaffle Cake:

- 2 tbsp. cocoa powder
- 2 tbsp. Swerve granulated sweetener
- 1 egg
- 1 tbsp. heavy whipping cream
- 1 tbsp. almond flour
- ¼ tsp. baking powder
- ½ tsp. vanilla extract

Cream Cheese Frosting:

- 2 tbsp. cream cheese
- 2 tsp. swerve confectioners
- 1/8 tsp. vanilla extract
- 1 tsp. heavy cream

Directions:

Chocolate Chaffle Cake:

1. Whisk cocoa powder, swerve, almond flour, and baking powder.
2. Stir in the vanilla extract and heavy whipping cream and mix well.
3. Pour in the egg and mix well. Be sure to scrape the sides of the bowl to get all of the ingredients mixed well.
4. Set aside for 3–4 minutes while the mini waffle maker heats up.
5. Ladle half of the waffle mixture into the waffle maker and cook for 4 minutes. While the second chaffle is cooking, create your frosting.

Cream Cheese Frosting:

1. Using a small microwave-safe bowl, stir in 2 tbsp. cream cheese. Heat up the cream cheese for 8 seconds to soften the cream cheese.
2. Pour in heavy whipping cream and vanilla extract and use a small hand mixer to mix well.
3. Stir in the confectioners, swerve, and use the hand mixer to incorporate and fluff the frosting.

Assembling Keto Chocolate Chaffle Cake:

1. Put one chocolate chaffle on a plate, top with a layer of frosting. You can spread it with a knife or use a pastry bag and pipe the frosting.
2. Place the second chocolate chaffle on top, then pipe the rest of the frosting on top.

Nutrition:

- **Calories**: 151
- **Protein**: 6 g
- **Fat**: 13 g
- **Carbohydrates**: 9 g

Preparation Time: 5 minutes

Cooking Time: 7 minutes

Servings: 2

Ingredients:

For Cake Layers:

- 1 tbsp. butter melted
- 1 tbsp. Golden Monk fruit sweetener
- 1 egg yolk
- 1/8 tsp. vanilla extract
- 1/8 tsp. Cake Batter Extract
- 3 tbsp. almond flour
- 1/8 tsp. baking powder
- 1 tbsp. chocolate chips sugar-free

Whipped Cream Frosting:

- 1 tsp. unflavored gelatin
- 4 tsp. Cold Water
- 1 Cup HWC
- 2 tbsp. Confectioners Sweetener

Directions:

Cake:

1. Mix all the ingredients and cook in a mini waffle iron for 4 minutes. Do it for each layer.

Whipped Cream Frosting Instructions:

1. Put your beaters and your mixing bowl in the freezer for about 15 minutes to allow them to cool.
2. Using a microwave-safe bowl, sprinkle the gelatin over the cold water. Stir, and allow to "bloom." This takes about 5 minutes.
3. Heat up the gelatin mixture for 10 seconds. It will become a liquid. Stir to make sure everything is dissolved.

4. Using a chilled mixing bowl, begin whipping the cream at a low speed. Add in the confectioner's sugar.

5. Adjust to higher speed and watch for good peaks to begin to form.

6. When its peak, switch back to a lower speed and slowly drizzle the melted liquid gelatin mixture in. Once it's in, switch back to a higher speed and continue to beat until it's reached stiff peaks.

7. Transfer into piping bags and pipe on your cake.

Nutrition:

- **Calories**: 171
- **Protein**: 4 g
- **Fat**: 16 g
- **Carbohydrates**: 11 g

Preparation Time: 5 minutes

Cooking Time: 7 minutes

Servings: 8

Ingredients:

Sweet Chaffle:

- 4 oz. cream cheese room temp
- 4 eggs
- 1 tbsp. melted butter
- 1 tsp. vanilla extract
- ½ tsp. cinnamon
- 1 tbsp. monk fruit sweetener
- 4 tbsp. coconut flour
- 1 tbsp. almond flour
- 1 ½ tsp. baking powder
- 1 tbsp. coconut shredded and unsweetened
- 1 tbsp. walnuts chopped

Italian Cream Frosting:

- 2 oz. cream cheese room temp
- 2 tbsp. butter room temp
- 2 tbsp. monk fruit sweetener or your favorite keto-approved sweetener
- ½ tsp. vanilla

Directions:

1. Using a medium-size blender, add cream cheese, eggs, melted butter, vanilla, sweetener, coconut flour, almond flour, and baking powder.
2. Mix the ingredients on high until it's smooth and creamy.
3. Set up the mini waffle maker.
4. Pour in the ingredients to the prepared waffle maker.
5. Cook for 3 minutes.
6. Remove and allow the chaffles to cool.

7. In a separate bowl, start to make the frosting by adding all the ingredients together. Stir until it's smooth and creamy.

8. Once the chaffles have completely cool, frost the cake.

Nutrition:

- **Calories:** 109
- **Fat:** 9.7 g
- **Protein:** 5.3 g
- **Carbohydrates:** 12 g

Preparation Time: 5 minutes

Cooking Time: 7 minutes

Servings: 2

Ingredients:

- 1 egg
- 2 tbsp. almond flour
- ½ tsp. coconut flour
- 1 tbsp. butter melted
- 1 tbsp. cream cheese room temp
- 20 drops Captain Cereal flavoring
- ¼ tsp. vanilla extract
- ¼ tsp. baking powder
- 1 tbsp. confectioners' sweetener
- 1/8 tsp. xanthan gum

Directions:

1. Set up the mini waffle maker.
2. Blend all of the ingredients until smooth. Set aside batter for a few minutes for the flour to absorb the liquid.
3. Pour in 3 tablespoons of batter into your waffle maker and cook it for about 2 ½ minutes.
4. Garnish with fresh whipped cream.

Nutrition:

- **Calories:** 154
- **Fat:** 11.2 g
- **Protein:** 4.6 g
- **Carbohydrates:** 6 g

Preparation Time: 5 minutes

Cooking Time: 7 minutes

Servings: 4

Ingredients:

German Chocolate Chaffle Cake:

- 2 eggs
- 1 tbsp. melted butter
- 1 tbsp. cream cheese softened to room temperature
- 2 tbsp. unsweetened cocoa powder
- 2 tbsp. almond flour
- 2 tsp. coconut flour
- 2 tbsp. Pyure granulated sweetener blend
- ½ tsp. baking powder
- ½ tsp. instant coffee granules dissolved in 1 tbsp. hot water
- ½ tsp. vanilla extract
- 2 pinches salt

German Chocolate Chaffle Cake Filling:

- 1 egg yolk
- ¼ cup heavy cream
- 2 tbsp. Pyure granulated sweetener blend
- 1 tbsp. butter
- ½ tsp. caramel or maple extract
- ¼ cup chopped pecans
- ¼ cup unsweetened flaked coconut
- 1 tsp. coconut flour

Directions:

Chaffle:

1. Set up mini Dash waffle iron until thoroughly hot.
2. Using a medium bowl, whisk all ingredients together until well combined.
3. Ladle heaping 2 tbsp. of batter into waffle iron, close, and cook 3-5 minutes, until done.
4. Put to a wire rack.
5. Repeat 3 times.

Filling:

1. Using a saucepan over medium heat, combine the egg yolk, heavy cream, butter, and sweetener.
2. Simmer gradually, constantly stirring for 6 minutes.
3. Pull away from heat and stir in extract, pecans, coconut flour, and flaked coconut.

Assembly:

1. Layout one-third of the filling in between each of 2 layers of chaffles and the remaining third on top chaffle and serve.

Nutrition:

- **Calories**: 271
- **Fat**: 23.7 g
- **Protein**: 7.6 g
- **Carbohydrates**: 8 g

Preparation Time: 5 minutes

Cooking Time: 7 minutes

Servings: 2

Ingredients:

Peanut Butter Chaffle:

- 2 tbsp. sugar-free Peanut Butter Powder
- 2 tbsp. Monk Fruit Confectioner's
- 1 egg
- ¼ tsp. baking powder
- 1 tbsp. heavy whipping cream
- ¼ tsp. Peanut Butter extract

Peanut Butter Frosting:

- 2 tbsp. Monk Fruit Confectioners
- 1 tbsp. butter softened and room temp
- 1 tbsp. sugar-free natural peanut butter or peanut butter powder
- 2 tbsp. cream cheese softened and room temp
- ¼ tsp. vanilla

Directions:

1. Whisk up the egg.
2. Mix in remaining ingredients the batter is smooth and creamy.
3. If you don't have the peanut butter extract, you can skip it. It does add a more intense peanut butter flavor that is absolutely wonderful and makes this extract worth investing in.
4. Fill in half the batter in a mini waffle maker and cook it for 2 to 3 minutes.
5. Incorporate sweetener, cream cheese, sugar-free natural peanut butter, and vanilla. Blend the frosting until everything is well incorporated.
6. Lay out the frosting on the waffle cake after it has completely cooled down to room temp.
7. Or you can pipe the frosting too!
8. Or you can heat the frosting and add a ½ tsp. of water to make it a peanut butter glaze; you can drizzle on your peanut butter chaffle too!

Nutrition:

- **Calories**: 144
- **Fat**: 7 g
- **Protein**: 5.5 g
- **Carbohydrates**: 11 g

Preparation Time: 5 minutes

Cooking Time: 7 minutes

Servings: 4

Ingredients:

Chaffle Cake:

- 2 eggs
- ¼ cup almond flour
- 1 tsp. coconut flour
- 2 tbsp. melted butter
- 2 tbsp. cream cheese room temp
- 20 drops Boston Cream extract
- ½ tsp. vanilla extract
- ½ tsp. baking powder
- 2 tbsp. swerve confectioners' sweetener or monk fruit
- ¼ tsp. Xanthan powder

Custard:

- ½ cup heavy whipping cream
- ½ tsp. vanilla extract
- 1 /2 tbsp. Swerve confectioners Sweetener
- 2 egg yolks
- 1/8 tsp. Xanthan gum

Ganache:

- 2 tbsp. heavy whipping cream
- 2 tbsp. unsweetened baking chocolate bar chopped
- 1 tbsp. Swerve Confectioners Sweetener

Directions:

1. Set up the mini waffle iron to make cake chaffles first.
2. Using a blender, mix all the cake ingredients and blend it on high until smooth and creamy.

3. On the stovetop, warm-up heavy whipping cream to a boil. While it's heating, whisk egg yolks and Swerve together in a separate small bowl.

4. When the cream is boiling, fill in half of it into the egg yolks. Ensure you are whisking it together while you pour in the mixture slowly.

5. Transfer the egg and cream mixture back into the stovetop pan into the rest of the cream and stir continuously for another 2-3 minutes.

6. Place the custard off the heat and whisk in your vanilla & xanthan gum. Then set it aside to cool and thicken.

7. Put ingredients for the ganache in a small bowl. Microwave for 20 seconds, stir. Repeat if needed. Careful not to overheat the ganache and burn it. Only do 20 seconds at a time until it's fully melted.

8. Serve your Boston cream pie Chaffle Cake and Enjoy!

Nutrition:

- **Calories**: 301
- **Fat**: 53.3 g
- **Protein**: 12.4 g
- **Carbohydrates**: 9 g

Preparation Time: 5 minutes

Cooking Time: 7 minutes

Servings: 6

Ingredients:

Chaffles:

- 2 eggs
- 1-ounce cream cheese softened to room temperature
- 2 tbsp. finely shredded unsweetened coconut
- 2 tbsp. Swerve
- 1 tbsp. melted butter
- ½ tsp. coconut extract
- ½ tsp. vanilla extract

Filling:

- 1/3 cup coconut milk
- 1/3 cup unsweetened almond milk
- 2 eggs yolks
- 2 tbsp. Swerve
- ¼ tsp. xanthan gum
- 2 tsp. butter
- Pinch salt
- ¼ cup finely shredded unsweetened coconut

Optional toppings:

- Sugar-free whipped cream
- 1 tbsp. thinly shredded unsweetened coconut toasted

Directions:

Chaffles:

1. Set up mini Dash waffle iron until thoroughly hot.
2. Incorporate all the chaffle ingredients together.

3. Ladle heaping 2 tablespoons of batter to waffle iron and cook until golden brown, and the waffle iron stops steaming, about 5 minutes.
4. Do it 3 times to make 4 chaffles. You only need 3 for the recipe.

For the Filling:

1. Warm-up coconut and almond milk in a small saucepan at medium-low heat. It must be steaming hot but not simmering.
2. Whisk egg yolks together lightly. While whisking the milk constantly, gradually drizzle the egg yolks into the milk.
3. Heat up constantly, stirring until the mixture thickens slightly. Do not boil. Whisk in the sweetener.
4. While constantly whisking, gradually sprinkle in the xanthan gum. Continue to cook for a minute.
5. Pull away from the heat and add the remaining ingredients.
6. Fill in coconut cream filling into a container, cover the surface with plastic wrap, and chill. The plastic wrap prevents skin from forming on the filling. The mixture will thicken as it cools.

Cake Assembly:

1. Spread 1/3 of the filling over each of 3 chaffles, stack them together to make a cake
2. Top with whipped cream and garnish with toasted coconut.

Nutrition:

- **Calories**: 157
- **Protein**: 5.1 g
- **Fat**: 14.1 g
- **Carbohydrates**: 9 g

Preparation Time: 5 minutes

Cooking Time: 7 minutes

Servings: 6

Ingredients:

Chocolate Chaffles:

- 1 egg
- 1-ounce cream cheese
- 1 tbsp. almond flour
- 1 tbsp. unsweetened cocoa powder
- 1 tbsp. erythritol sweeteners blends such as Swerve, Pyure or Lakanto
- ½ tsp. vanilla extract
- ¼ tsp. instant coffee powder

Coconut Filling:

- 1 ½ tsp. coconut oil melted
- 1 tbsp. heavy cream
- ¼ cup unsweetened finely shredded coconut
- 2 ounces cream cheese
- 1 tbsp. confectioner's sweetener such as Swerve
- ¼ tsp. vanilla extract
- 14 whole almonds

Directions:

For the Chaffles:

1. Set up a mini-Dash waffle iron until thoroughly hot.
2. Whisk all chaffle ingredients together until well combined.
3. Fill in half of the batter into the waffle iron.
4. Cook 4 minutes, until done. Put to a wire rack.
5. Do it again for the second chaffle.

For the Filling:

1. Soften cream to room temperature or warm in the microwave for 10 seconds.

2. Stir in all ingredients to a bowl and mix until smooth and well-combined.

Assemble:

1. Layout half the filling on one chaffle and drizzle 7 almonds evenly on top of the filling.

2. Do with the second chaffle and stack together.

Nutrition:

- **Calories**: 130
- **Protein**: 3 g
- **Fat**: 10.6 g
- **Carbohydrates**: 8 g

Preparation Time: 5 minutes

Cooking Time: 7 minutes

Servings: 2

Ingredients:

Keto Sugar Cookie:

- 1 tbsp. butter melted
- 1 tbsp. sweetener
- 1 egg yolk
- 1/8 tsp. vanilla extract
- 1/8 tsp. Cake Batter Extract
- 3 T almond flour
- 1/8 tsp. baking powder

Icing:

- 1 tbsp. Confectioners Sweetener
- ¼ tsp. vanilla extract
- 1-2 tsp. water

Sprinkles

- 1 T Granular Sweetener blend with 1 drop food coloring.

Directions:

1. Stir all ingredients together. Let rest for 5 min.
2. Stir again.
3. Refrigerate for 15 minutes.
4. Put ½ of the dough in the pumpkin waffle maker.
5. Cook 4 minutes.
6. Repeat. Let cool.
7. Add icing and sprinkles, if desired.

Nutrition:

- **Calories:** 151
- **Protein:** 6 g
- **Fat:** 13 g
- **Carbohydrates:** 9 g

Preparation Time: 5 minutes

Cooking Time: 7 minutes

Servings: 2

Ingredients:

Chaffle:

- 1 egg
- 1 tbsp. black cocoa
- 1 tbsp. monk fruit confectioner's blend
- ¼ tsp. baking powder
- 2 tbsp. cream cheese room temp
- 1 tbsp. mayonnaise
- ¼ tsp. instant coffee powder
- pinch salt
- 1 tsp. vanilla

Frosting:

- 2 tbsp. monk fruit confectioners
- 2 tbsp. cream cheese softened and room temp
- ¼ tsp. clear vanilla

Directions:

1. In a small bowl, whip up the egg.
2. Add the remaining ingredients and mix well until the batter is smooth and creamy.
3. Divide the batter into 3 and pour each in a mini waffle maker and cook it for 2 ½ to 3 minutes until it's fully cooked.
4. In a separate small bowl, add the sweetener, cream cheese, and vanilla. Mix the frosting until everything is well incorporated.
5. Spread the frosting on the waffle cake after it has completely cooled down to room temperature.

Nutrition:

- **Calories:** 159
- **Protein:** 8 g
- **Fat:** 11 g
- **Carbohydrates:** 9 g

Preparation Time: 5 minutes

Cooking Time: 7 minutes

Servings: 2

Ingredients:

Chaffles:

- 1 egg
- 1-ounce cream cheese softened to room temperature
- 2 tsp. melted butter
- 1 tbsp. Swerve Brown sweetener
- 1 tbsp. almond flour
- 2 tsp. coconut flour
- ¼ tsp. baking powder
- 3/4 tsp. ground ginger
- ½ tsp. ground cinnamon
- Generous dash ground nutmeg
- Generous dash ground clove

Icing:

- 2 tbsp. Swerve or Lakanto
- 1 ½ tsp. heavy cream
- 1/8 tsp. maple extract

Directions:

1. Prep a mini-Dash waffle iron until thoroughly hot.
2. Whisk all the chaffle ingredients together in a small bowl until smooth.
3. Ladle heaping 2 tbsp. of batter to waffle iron and cook until done about 4 minutes.
4. Do it again to make 2 chaffles. Let cool on the wire rack.

Maple Icing:

1. Whisk sweetener, heavy cream, and maple extract until smooth.
2. Pour enough water to thin to a spreadable consistency.
3. Layout the icing on each chaffle and sprinkle with additional ground cinnamon, if desired.

Nutrition:

- **Calories**: 161
- **Fat**: 12.5 g
- **Protein**: 5.2 g
- **Carbohydrates**: 5 g

Preparation Time: 5 minutes

Cooking Time: 7 minutes

Servings: 2

Ingredients:

- 1 large Egg
- ½ c. Mozzarella cheese shredded
- ½ tsp. vanilla extract
- 2 tbsp. swerve brown
- ½ tbsp. Psyllium Husk Powder optional
- ¼ tsp. baking powder
- Pinch pink salt
- ¼ Lily's Original Dark Chocolate Bar
- 2 tbsp. Keto Marshmallow Crème Fluff Recipe

Directions:

Keto Marshmallow Crème Fluff:

1. Whip the egg until creamy.
2. Stir in vanilla and Swerve Brown; mix well.
3. Drizzle the shredded cheese and blend.
4. Mix in Psyllium Husk Powder, baking powder, and salt.
5. Mix until well incorporated, set aside for 3–4 minutes.
6. Prep your waffle maker to preheat.
7. Lay ½ batter on the waffle maker and cook 3–4 minutes.
8. Take it out and set it on a cooling rack.
9. Cook the second half of batter same, then remove to cool.
10. When cool, assemble the chaffles with the marshmallow fluff and chocolate:
11. With 2 tbsp. marshmallow and ¼ bar of Lily's Chocolate.

Nutrition:

- **Fat:** 8.1 g
- **Protein:** 8.3 g
- **Carbohydrates:** 7 g

Preparation Time: 5 minutes

Cooking Time: 7 minutes

Servings: 3

Ingredients:

- 1 egg
- ½ cup mozzarella cheese
- ½ tsp. pumpkin pie spice
- 1 tbsp. pumpkin solid packed with no sugar added

Optional Cream Cheese Frosting:

- 2 tbsp. cream cheese softened and room temperature
- 2 tbsp. monk fruit confectioners blend or your favorite keto-friendly sweetener
- ½ tsp. clear vanilla extract

Directions:

1. Heat up the mini waffle maker.
2. Whisk the egg.
3. Drizzle cheese, pumpkin pie spice, and the pumpkin.
4. Mix well.
5. Pour ½ of the mixture into the mini waffle maker and cook it for at least 3 to 4 minutes until it's golden brown.
6. While it's cooking, mix in all of the cream cheese frosting ingredients in a bowl and mix it until it's smooth and creamy.
7. Pour in cream cheese frosting to the hot chaffle and serve it immediately.

Nutrition:

- **Calories:** 84
- **Fat:** 4.5 g
- **Protein:** 6.1 g
- **Carbohydrates:** 5 g

Preparation Time: 5 minutes

Cooking Time: 7 minutes

Servings: 4

Ingredients:

- 2 tbsp. butter melted (cooled)
- 2 ounces cream cheese softened
- 2 large eggs room temp
- 1 tsp. vanilla extract
- ½ tsp. Vanilla Cupcake Extract (optional)
- ¼ cup Lakanto Confectioners
- Pinch pink salt
- ¼ cup almond flour
- 2 tbsp. coconut flour
- 1 tsp. baking powder

Directions:

1. Heat up the Corndog Maker.
2. Cook the butter and let it cool a minute.
3. Whip the eggs into the butter until creamy.
4. Stir in vanilla, extract, sweetener, salt, and then blend well.
5. Mix in almond flour, coconut flour, and baking powder.
6. Blend until well incorporated.
7. Ladle 2 tbsp. batter to each well and spread across evenly.
8. Cook for 4 minutes.
9. Take it out and chill on a rack.

Nutrition:

- **Calories:** 152
- **Fat:** 9 g
- **Protein:** 6.1 g
- **Carbohydrates:** 9 g

Preparation Time: 5 minutes

Cooking Time: 7 minutes

Servings: 6

Ingredients:

Chaffles:

- 1 egg
- 1 oz. cream cheese at room temp
- 1 tbsp. melted butter or coconut oil
- 1 tbsp. unsweetened cocoa powder or raw cacao
- 2 tbsp. powdered sweeteners such as Swerve or Lakanto
- 1 tbsp. almond flour
- 2 tsp. coconut flour
- ¼ tsp. baking powder
- 1 tsp. instant coffee granules
- ¼ tsp. vanilla extract

Filling:

- 2 tbsp. butter at room temp
- 2-3 tbsp. Swerve
- ¼ tsp. vanilla extract
- 1/8 tsp. peppermint extract

Optional Toppings:
- Sugar-free starlight mints

Directions:

For the Mocha Chaffles:

1. Set up a mini-Dash waffle iron until thoroughly hot.
2. Whisk all chaffle ingredients together in a small bowl until smooth.
3. Ladle heaping 2 tbsp. of batter to waffle iron and cook until done about 4 minutes.
4. Do it again to make 3 chaffles. Let cool on the wire rack.

For the Buttercream Frosting:

1. In a small bowl with a hand mixer, beat the butter and sweetener until smooth.
2. Add the heavy cream and vanilla extract and beat at high speed for about 4 minutes, until light and fluffy.
3. Spread frosting on each chaffle and garnish with sugar-free starlight mints, if desired.

Nutrition:

- **Calories**: 96
- **Protein**: 1.9 g
- **Fat**: 8.9 g
- **Carbohydrates**: 11 g

Preparation Time: 15 minutes

Cooking Time: 28 minutes

Servings: 4

Ingredients:

For the Chaffles:

- 2 eggs, beaten
- ½ cup finely grated Parmesan cheese
- 2 oz. cream cheese, softened
- 2 drops red food coloring
- 1 tsp. vanilla extract

For the Frosting:

- 3 tbsp. cream cheese, softened
- 1 tbsp. sugar-free maple syrup
- ¼ tsp. vanilla extract

Directions:

For the Chaffles:

1. Preheat the waffle iron.
2. Incorporate all the ingredients for the chaffles.
3. Open the iron and add a quarter of the mixture. Close and cook until crispy, 7 minutes.
4. Transfer the chaffle to a plate and make 3 more chaffles with the remaining batter.

For the Frosting:

1. In a medium bowl, using a hand mixer, whisk the cream cheese, maple syrup, and vanilla extract until smooth.
2. Assemble the chaffles with the frosting to make the cake.
3. Slice and serve.

Nutrition:

- **Calories:** 147
- **Fat:** 9.86 g
- **Protein:** 8.57 g
- **Carbohydrates:** 12 g

Preparation Time: 10 minutes

Cooking Time: 28 minutes

Servings: 4

Ingredients:

For the Chaffles:

- 2 eggs, beaten
- ½ cup finely grated Swiss cheese
- 2 oz. cream cheese, softened
- ½ tsp. lemon extract
- 20 drops cake batter extract

For the Frosting:

- ½ cup heavy cream
- 1 tbsp. sugar-free maple syrup
- ¼ tsp. lemon extract

Directions:

For the Chaffles:

1. Preheat the waffle iron.
2. Incorporate all the ingredients for the chaffles.
3. Open the iron and add a quarter of the mixture. Close and cook until crispy, 7 minutes.
4. Transfer the chaffle to a plate and make 3 more chaffles with the remaining batter.

For the Frosting:

1. Using a hand mixer, a medium bowl, beat the heavy cream, maple syrup, and lemon extract until fluffy.
2. Assemble the chaffles with the frosting to make the cake.
3. Slice and serve.

Nutrition:

- **Calories:** 176
- **Fat:** 15.18 g
- **Protein:** 7.63 g
- **Carbohydrates:** 11 g

Preparation Time: 20 minutes

Cooking Time: 28 minutes

Servings: 4

Ingredients:

For the Chaffles:

- 1 egg, beaten
- 1/3 cup finely grated mozzarella cheese
- 1 tbsp. almond flour
- 2 tbsp. almond butter
- 1 tbsp. swerve confectioner's sugar
- ½ tsp. vanilla extract

For the Chocolate Butter Frosting:

- 1½ cups butter, room temperature
- 1 cup unsweetened cocoa powder
- ½ cup almond milk
- 5 cups swerve confectioner's sugar
- 2 tsp. vanilla extract

Directions:

For the Chaffles:

1. Preheat the waffle iron.
2. In a medium bowl, mix the egg, mozzarella cheese, almond flour, almond butter, swerve confectioner's sugar, and vanilla extract.
3. Open the iron and add a quarter of the mixture. Close and cook until crispy, 7 minutes.
4. Transfer the chaffle to a plate and make 3 more chaffles with the remaining batter.

For the Frosting:

1. Whisk butter and cocoa powder until smooth.
2. Gradually, whisk in the almond milk and swerve confectioner's sugar until smooth.
3. Add the vanilla extract and mix well.

4. Assemble the chaffles with the frosting to make the cake.

5. Slice and serve.

Nutrition:

- **Calories**: 838
- **Fat**: 85.35 g
- **Protein**: 13.5 g
- **Carbohydrates**: 16 g

Preparation Time: 25 minutes

Cooking Time: 28 minutes

Servings: 4

Ingredients:

For the Custard Filling:

- 4 egg yolks, beaten
- 1 tbsp. erythritol
- ¼ tsp. xanthan gum
- 1 cup heavy cream
- 1 tbsp. vanilla extract

For the Chaffles:

- 2 eggs, beaten
- 2 tbsp. cream cheese, softened
- 1 cup finely grated Monterey Jack cheese
- 1 tsp. vanilla extract
- 1 tbsp. heavy cream
- 1 tbsp. coconut flour
- ½ tsp. baking powder
- ½ tsp. ground cinnamon
- ¼ tsp. erythritol

Directions:

For the Custard Filling:

1. Whisk egg yolks with the erythritol. Mix in the xanthan gum until smooth.
2. Pour the heavy cream into a medium saucepan and simmer over low heat. Pour the mixture into the egg mixture while whisking vigorously until well mixed.
3. Transfer the mixture to the saucepan and continue whisking while cooking over low heat until thickened, 20 to 30 seconds. Put the heat off and stir in the vanilla extract.
4. Strain the custard through a fine mesh into a bowl. Cover the bowl with plastic wrap.
5. Refrigerate for 1 hour.

For the Chaffles:

1. After 1 hour, preheat the waffle iron.
2. Incorporate all the ingredients for the chaffles.
3. Open the iron and add a quarter of the mixture. Close and cook until crispy, 7 minutes.
4. Transfer the chaffle to a plate and make 3 more with the remaining batter.
5. To serve:
6. Spread the custard filling between two chaffle quarters, sandwich, and enjoy!

Nutrition:

- **Calories**: 239
- **Fat**: 21.25 g
- **Protein**: 6.73 g
- **Carbohydrates**: 15 g

Preparation Time: 20 minutes

Cooking Time: 28 minutes

Servings: 4

Ingredients:

For the Chaffles:

- 2 eggs, beaten
- 3 tbsp. cream cheese, softened
- ½ cup finely grated Gouda cheese
- 1 tsp. vanilla extract
- ¼ tsp. erythritol

For the Coffee Syrup:

- 2 tbsp. strong coffee, room temperature
- 3 tbsp. sugar-free maple syrup

For the Filling:

- ¼ cup heavy cream
- 2 tsp. vanilla extract
- ¼ tsp. erythritol
- 4 tbsp. mascarpone cheese, room temperature
- 1 tbsp. cream cheese, softened

For Dusting:
- ½ tsp. unsweetened cocoa powder

Directions:

For the Chaffles:

1. Preheat the waffle iron.
2. Incorporate all the ingredients for the chaffles.
3. Open the iron and add a quarter of the mixture. Close and cook until crispy, 7 minutes.
4. Transfer the chaffle to a plate and make 3 more with the remaining batter.

For the Coffee Syrup:

1. In a small bowl, mix the coffee and maple syrup. Set aside.
2. For the filling:
3. Beat the heavy cream, vanilla, and erythritol in a medium bowl using an electric hand mixer until stiff peak forms.
4. Whisk mascarpone cheese and cream cheese until well combined. Add the heavy cream mixture and fold in. Spoon the mixture into a piping bag.

To Assemble:

1. Spoon 1 tbsp. of the coffee syrup on one chaffle and pipe some of the cream cheese mixture on top. Cover with another chaffle and continue the assembling process.
2. Generously dust with cocoa powder and refrigerate overnight.
3. When ready to enjoy, slice, and serve.

Nutrition:

- **Calories**: 208
- **Fat**: 15.91 g
- **Protein**: 10.1 g
- **Carbohydrates**: 19 g

Preparation Time: 15 minutes

Cooking Time: 28 minutes

Servings: 4

Ingredients:

For the Chaffles:

- 2 eggs, beaten
- 2 tbsp. cream cheese, softened
- 1 cup finely grated Monterey Jack cheese
- 2 tbsp. coconut flour
- ¼ tsp. baking powder
- 1 tbsp. unsweetened shredded coconut
- 1 tbsp. walnuts, chopped

For the Frosting:

- ¼ cup unsalted butter, room temperature
- 3 tbsp. almond milk
- 1 tsp. mint extract
- 2 drops green food coloring
- 3 cups swerve confectioner's sugar

Directions:

For the Chaffles:

1. Preheat the waffle iron.
2. Incorporate all the ingredients for the chaffles.
3. Open the iron and add a quarter of the mixture. Close and cook until crispy, 7 minutes.
4. Transfer the chaffle to a plate and make 3 more with the remaining batter.

For the Frosting:

1. In a medium bowl, cream the butter using an electric hand mixer until smooth.
2. Gradually mix in the almond milk until smooth.
3. Add the mint extract and green food coloring; whisk until well combined.

4. Finally, mix in the swerve confectioner's sugar a cup at a time until smooth.

5. Layer the chaffles with the frosting.

6. Slice and serve afterward.

Nutrition:

- **Calories**: 141
- **Fat**: 13.13 g
- **Protein**: 4.31 g
- **Carbohydrates**: 5 g

Preparation Time: 15 minutes

Cooking Time: 28 minutes

Servings: 4

Ingredients:

For the Cinnamon Roll Chaffles:

- ½ cup finely grated mozzarella cheese
- 1 egg, beaten
- 1 tsp. cinnamon powder
- 1 tbsp. almond flour
- 1 tsp. erythritol

For the Cinnamon Roll Swirl:

- 1 tbsp. butter
- 1 tsp. cinnamon powder
- 2 tsp. erythritol

For the Cinnamon Roll Glaze:

- 1 tbsp. butter, melted
- 1 tbsp. cream cheese, melted
- ¼ tsp. vanilla extract
- 2 tsp. swerve confectioner's sugar

Directions:

1. Preheat the waffle iron.
2. Incorporate all the ingredients for the chaffles. Set aside.
3. In another bowl, mix all the ingredients for the cinnamon roll swirl.
4. Open the iron and lightly grease with cooking spray. Add a quarter of the chaffle mixture and top with the cinnamon roll swirl mixture.
5. Cook for 7 minutes.
6. Transfer the chaffle to a plate and make 3 more with the remaining ingredients.
7. Meanwhile, in a small bowl, whisk the glaze ingredients until smooth.
8. Drizzle the glaze over the chaffles when they are ready and serve afterward.

Nutrition:

- **Calories**: 112
- **Fat**: 10.2 g
- **Protein**: 3.38 g
- **Carbohydrates**: 11 g

Preparation Time: 15 minutes

Cooking Time: 36 minutes

Servings: 4

Ingredients:

For the Chaffles:

- 2 eggs, beaten
- ¼ cup finely grated Gruyere cheese
- 2 tbsp. heavy cream
- 1 tbsp. coconut flour
- 2 tbsp. cream cheese, softened
- 3 tbsp. unsweetened cocoa powder
- 2 tsp. vanilla extract
- A pinch salt

For the Chocolate Sauce:

- 1/3 cup + 1 tbsp. heavy cream
- 1 ½ oz. unsweetened baking chocolate, chopped
- 1 ½ tsp. sugar-free maple syrup
- 1 ½ tsp. vanilla extract

Directions:

For the Chaffles:

1. Preheat the waffle iron.
2. Incorporate all the ingredients for the chaffles.
3. Open the iron and add a quarter of the mixture. Close and cook until crispy, 7 minutes.
4. Transfer the chaffle to a plate and make 3 more with the remaining batter.

For the Chocolate Sauce:

1. Pour the heavy cream into a saucepan and simmer over low heat, 3 minutes.
2. Put the heat off and stir in the chocolate. Allow melting for a few minutes and stir until fully melted, 5 minutes.

3. Mix in the maple syrup and vanilla extract.

4. Assemble the chaffles in layers with the chocolate sauce sandwiched between each layer.

5. Slice and serve immediately.

Nutrition:

- **Calories:** 172
- **Fat:** 13.57 g
- **Protein:** 5.76 g
- **Carbohydrates:** 19 g

Preparation Time: 10 minutes

Cooking Time: 14 minutes

Servings: 2

Ingredients:

- 1 egg, beaten
- ½ cup finely grated mozzarella cheese
- ¼ cup almond flour
- 2 tbsp. swerve confectioner's sugar
- 1/8 tsp. xanthan gum
- Low-carb ice cream (your flavor's choice) for serving

Directions:

1. Preheat the waffle iron.
2. Incorporate all the ingredients except the ice cream.
3. Open the iron and add half of the mixture. Close and cook until crispy, 7 minutes.
4. Transfer the chaffle to a plate and make a second one with the remaining batter.
5. On each chaffle, add a scoop of low-carb ice cream, fold into half-moons and enjoy.

Nutrition:

- **Calories:** 89
- **Fat:** 6.48 g
- **Protein:** 5.91 g
- **Carbohydrates:** 18 g

Preparation Time: 10 minutes

Cooking Time: 28 minutes

Servings: 4

Ingredients:

- 1 egg, beaten
- ½ cup finely grated mozzarella cheese
- 1 tbsp. almond flour
- ¼ tsp. baking powder
- 2 drops cake batter extract
- 1 cup cream cheese, softened
- 1 cup fresh strawberries, sliced
- 1 tbsp. sugar-free maple syrup

Directions:

1. Preheat a waffle bowl maker and grease lightly with cooking spray.
2. Meanwhile, in a medium bowl, whisk all the ingredients except the cream cheese and strawberries.
3. Open the iron, pour in half of the mixture, cover, and cook until crispy, 6 to 7 minutes.
4. Remove the chaffle bowl onto a plate and set it aside.
5. Make a second chaffle bowl with the remaining batter.
6. To serve, divide the cream cheese into the chaffle bowls and top with the strawberries.
7. Drizzle the filling with the maple syrup and serve.

Nutrition:

- **Calories**: 235
- **Fat**: 20.62 g
- **Protein**: 7.51 g
- **Carbohydrates**: 14 g

Preparation Time: 13 minutes

Cooking Time: 10 minutes

Servings: 3

Ingredients:

- Italian cream frosting
- 4 tbsp. Cream cheese
- 2 tbsp. butter
- ½ tsp. vanilla
- 2 tbsp. Monk fruit sweetener
- Chaffle
- 4 egg
- ½ cup Mozzarella cheese
- 1 tbsp. almond flour
- 4 tbsp. coconut flour
- 1 tbsp. Monk fruit sweetener
- 1 tsp. vanilla extract
- 1 ½ tsp. baking powder
- ½ tsp. cinnamon powder
- 1 tbsp. (melted) butter
- 1 tsp. coconut (shredded)
- 1 tsp. walnuts (chopped)

Directions:

1. Prepare a mix in a heated pan containing eggs, baking powder, almond flour, butter, coconut flour, vanilla, sweetener, and cream cheese. Stir into a thick creamy paste.
2. Preheat and grease the waffle maker. Pour the mixture into the lower side of the waffle maker and spread evenly. Heat the mixtures to a crunchy form for 5 minutes. Repeat the process for the remaining mixture.
3. Put the heat off and allow the chaffle to cool a bit. Stack up the chaffles with pudding into a single-row cake and garnish with shredded coconut and walnuts. Serve hot and enjoy the crispy taste.

Nutrition:

- **Calories:** 134
- **Protein:** 8 g
- **Fat:** 13 g
- **Carbohydrates:** 11 g

Preparation Time: 10 minutes

Cooking Time: 38 minutes

Servings: 4

Ingredients:

For the Chaffles:

- 1 egg, beaten
- ½ cup finely shredded cheddar cheese
- 1 tsp. almond flour
- 1 tsp. sour cream

For the Raspberry Syrup:

- 1 cup fresh raspberries
- ¼ cup swerve sugar
- ¼ cup water
- 1 tsp. vanilla extract

Directions:

For the Chaffles:

1. Preheat the waffle iron.
2. Incorporate egg, cheddar cheese, almond flour, and sour cream.
3. Open the iron, pour in half of the mixture, cover, and cook until crispy, 7 minutes.
4. Remove the chaffle onto a plate and make another with the remaining batter.

For the Raspberry Syrup:

1. Meanwhile, add the raspberries, swerve sugar, water, and vanilla extract to a medium pot. Adjust to low heat and cook until the raspberries soften and sugar becomes syrupy. Occasionally stir while mashing the raspberries as you go. Turn the heat off when your desired consistency is achieved and set aside to cool.
2. Drizzle some syrup on the chaffles and enjoy when ready.

Nutrition:

- **Calories:** 105
- **Fat:** 7.11 g
- **Protein:** 5.83 g
- **Carbohydrates:** 19 g

284. Chaffle Cannoli

Preparation Time: 15 minutes

Cooking Time: 28 minutes

Servings: 4

Ingredients:

For the Chaffles:

- 1 large egg
- 1 egg yolk
- 3 tbsp. butter, melted
- 1 tbsp. swerve confectioner's
- 1 cup finely grated Parmesan cheese
- 2 tbsp. finely grated mozzarella cheese

For the Cannoli Filling:

- ½ cup ricotta cheese
- 2 tbsp. swerve confectioner's sugar
- 1 tsp. vanilla extract
- 2 tbsp. unsweetened chocolate chips for garnishing

Directions:

1. Preheat the waffle iron.
2. Incorporate all the ingredients for the chaffles.
3. Open the iron, pour in a quarter of the mixture, cover, and cook until crispy, 7 minutes.
4. Remove the chaffle onto a plate and make 3 more with the remaining batter.
5. Meanwhile, for the cannoli filling:
6. Beat the ricotta cheese and swerve the confectioner's sugar until smooth. Mix in the vanilla.
7. On each chaffle, spread some of the fillings and wrap it over.
8. Garnish the creamy ends with some chocolate chips.
9. Serve immediately.

Nutrition:

- **Calories:** 308
- **Fat:** 25.05 g
- **Protein:** 15.18 g
- **Carbohydrates:** 21 g

Preparation Time: 10 minutes

Cooking Time: 28 minutes

Servings: 4

Ingredients:

- 1 egg, beaten
- ½ cup finely grated mozzarella cheese
- 1 tbsp. cream cheese, softened
- 1 tbsp. sugar-free maple syrup + extra for topping
- ½ cup blueberries
- ¼ tsp. vanilla extract

Directions:

1. Preheat the waffle iron.
2. Incorporate all the ingredients.
3. Open the iron, lightly grease with cooking spray, and pour in a quarter of the mixture.
4. Close the iron and cook until golden brown and crispy, 7 minutes.
5. Remove the chaffle onto a plate and set it aside.
6. Make the remaining chaffles with the remaining mixture.
7. Drizzle the chaffles with maple syrup and serve afterward.

Nutrition:

- **Calories:** 137
- **Fat:** 9.07 g
- **Protein:** 9.59 g
- **Carbohydrates:** 8 g

Preparation Time: 15 minutes

Cooking Time: 14 minutes

Servings: 2

Ingredients:

For the Chaffles:

- 2 tbsp. sugar-free peanut butter powder
- 2 tbsp. maple (sugar-free) syrup
- 1 egg, beaten
- ¼ cup finely grated mozzarella cheese
- ¼ tsp. baking powder
- ¼ tsp. almond butter
- ¼ tsp. peanut butter extract
- 1 tbsp. softened cream cheese

For the Frosting:

- ½ cup almond flour
- 1 cup peanut butter
- 3 tbsp. almond milk
- ½ tsp. vanilla extract
- ½ cup maple (sugar-free) syrup

Directions:

1. Preheat the waffle iron.
2. Incorporate all the ingredients until smooth.
3. Open the iron and pour in half of the mixture.
4. Close the iron and cook until crispy, 6 to 7 minutes.
5. Remove the chaffle onto a plate and set it aside.
6. Make a second chaffle with the remaining batter.
7. While the chaffles cool, make the frosting.
8. Pour the almond flour in a medium saucepan and stir-fry over medium heat until golden.

9. Transfer the almond flour to a blender and top with the remaining frosting ingredients. Process until smooth.

10. Spread the frosting on the chaffles and serve afterward.

Nutrition:

- **Calories**: 239
- **Fat**: 15.48 g
- **Protein**: 7.52 g
- **Carbohydrates**: 9 g

Preparation Time: 12 minutes

Cooking Time: 30 minutes

Servings: 4

Ingredients:

For the Chaffles:

- 2 eggs, beaten
- 1 tbsp. unsweetened cocoa powder
- 1 tbsp. erythritol
- 1 cup finely grated mozzarella cheese

For the Topping:

- 3 tbsp. unsweetened chocolate, chopped
- 3 tbsp. unsalted butter
- ½ cup swerve sugar

Low-Carb Ice Cream for Topping:

- 1 cup whipped cream for topping
- 3 tbsp. sugar-free caramel sauce

Directions:

For the Chaffles:

1. Preheat the waffle iron.
2. Meanwhile, in a medium bowl, mix all the ingredients for the chaffles.
3. Open the iron, pour in a quarter of the mixture, cover, and cook until crispy, 7 minutes.
4. Remove the chaffle onto a plate and make 3 more with the remaining batter.
5. Plate and set aside.

For the Topping:

1. Meanwhile, melt the chocolate and butter in a medium saucepan with occasional stirring, 2 minutes.

To Serve:

1. Divide the chaffles into wedges and top with the ice cream, whipped cream, and swirl the chocolate sauce and caramel sauce on top.

2. Serve immediately.

Nutrition:

- **Calories**: 165
- **Fat**: 11.39 g
- **Protein**: 12.79 g
- **Carbohydrates**: 9 g

Preparation Time: 15 minutes

Cooking Time: 36 minutes

Servings: 4

Ingredients:

For the Chaffles:

- 2 eggs, beaten
- 1 cup finely grated mozzarella cheese

For the Topping:

- 1 ½ cups blackberries
- 1 lemon, 1 tsp. zest and 2 tbsp. juice
- 1 tbsp. erythritol
- 4 slices Brie cheese

Directions:

For the Chaffles:

1. Preheat the waffle iron.
2. Meanwhile, in a medium bowl, mix the eggs and mozzarella cheese.
3. Open the iron, pour in a quarter of the mixture, cover, and cook until crispy, 7 minutes.
4. Remove the chaffle onto a plate and make 3 more with the remaining batter.
5. Plate and set aside.

For the Topping:

1. Preheat the oven to 350 F and line a baking sheet with parchment paper.
2. In a medium pot, add the blackberries, lemon zest, lemon juice, and erythritol. Cook until the blackberries break and the sauce thickens, 5 minutes. Turn the heat off.
3. Arrange the chaffles on the baking sheet and place two Brie cheese slices on each. Top with blackberry mixture and transfer the baking sheet to the oven.
4. Bake until the cheese melts, 2 to 3 minutes.
5. Remove from the oven, allow cooling, and serve afterward.

Nutrition:

- **Calories**: 576
- **Fat**: 42.22 g
- **Protein**: 42.35 g
- **Carbohydrates**: 16 g

Preparation Time: 60 minutes

Cooking Time: 12 minutes

Servings: 2

Ingredients:

- Banana pudding
- 1 large egg yolk
- ½ tsp. Xanthan gum
- ½ tsp. banana extract
- A pinch salt
- 3 tbsp. powdered sweetener:
- ½ cup Heavy Whipping Cream
- Banana chaffing
- 2 tbsp. cream cheese
- ¼ cup Mozzarella cheese
- 2 tbsp. sweetener
- 1 tsp. baking powder
- 1 tsp. banana extract
- 1 egg
- 4 tbsp. almond flour:

Directions:

1. Prepare a mix in a heated pan containing egg yolk, heavy cream, and powdered sweetener, all whisked together to a viscose mixture, then allow simmering for 1 minute. Add the gum and stir again vigorously.
2. Put off the heat, and add in the banana extract and salt to taste, then mix. Transfer the mixture into a glass and cool the pudding. Preheat and grease the waffle maker. Prepare a mix of all the ingredients in a mixing bowl. Pour the mixture into a large-sized waffle maker and spread evenly.
3. Heat the mixtures to a crunchy form for 5 minutes. Repeat the process for the remaining mixture. Put the heat off and allow the chaffle to cool a bit. Stack up the chaffles with pudding into a single-row cake. Serve hot and enjoy the crispy taste.

Nutrition:

- **Calories:** 159
- **Protein:** 6 g
- **Fat:** 11 g
- **Carbohydrates:** 15 g

Preparation Time: 12 minutes

Cooking Time: 6 minutes

Servings: 2

Ingredients:

- Cream cheese frosting
- ½ cup cream cheese
- 1 tsp. vanilla extract
- 2 tbsp. Heavy Whipping Cream
- ¼ cup powdered sweetener
- Carrot Chaffle Cake
- ½ cup carrot (shredded)
- ¾ cup almond flour
- 1 tsp. baking powder
- 1 egg
- 2 tbsp. butter (melted)
- 1 tbsp. walnuts (chopped)
- 2 tbsp. cinnamon powder:
- 1 tsp. pumpkin sauce:

Directions:

1. Prepare a mix containing all the ingredients and mix evenly to obtain a homogenous mixture. Preheat and grease the waffle maker.
2. Prepare a mix of all the ingredients in a mixing bowl. Pour the mixture into the lower side of the waffle maker and spread evenly. Heat the mixtures to a crunchy form for 5 minutes. Repeat the process for the remaining mixture.
3. Put the heat off and allow the chaffle to cool a bit. Stack up the chaffles with pudding into a single-row cake. Serve hot and enjoy the crispy taste.

Nutrition:

- **Calories**: 151
- **Protein**: 6 g
- **Fat**: 13 g
- **Carbohydrates**: 19 g

291. Pecan Pie Cake Chaffle

Preparation Time: 26 minutes

Cooking Time: 18 minutes

Servings: 2

Ingredients:

- Pecan Pie Filling
- 2 tbsp. butter
- 2 tbsp. chopped pecan
- 2 tbsp. maple syrup
- A pinch salt
- 1 tbsp. Sukrin Gold
- 2 tbsp. Heavy Whipping Cream
- 2 large egg yolk
- Pecan Pie Chaffle
- 1 egg
- ½ tbsp. maple extract
- 1 tbsp. Sukrin Gold
- 2 tbsp. chopped Pecan
- 2 tbsp. cream cheese
- 4 tbsp. almond flour
- ½ tbsp. baking powder

Directions:

1. Prepare a mix in a low heated saucepan containing heavy whipping cream, syrups, butter, and sweetener. Mix all ingredients together into a thick creamy paste. Put off the heat and pour in the egg yolks, then place on heat again and mix.
2. Pour in the chopped Pecans with a pinch of salt to taste, and then allow simmering to thicken. Put off the heat. For the chaffles, prepare the mix of all ingredients into a blender and blend, except for the pecans. Add in the chopped pecans and stir.

3. Preheat and grease the waffle maker. Pour the mixture into the lower side of the waffle maker and spread evenly. Heat the mixtures to a crunchy form for 5 minutes. Repeat the process for the remaining mixture.

4. Put the heat off and allow the chaffle to cool a bit. Stack up the chaffles into a single-row cake and garnish 1/3 of the pecan pie filling earlier prepared on the chaffle. Serve hot and enjoy the crispy taste.

Nutrition:

- **Calories:** 174
- **Protein:** 11 g
- **Fat:** 20 g
- **Carbohydrates:** 19 g

Preparation Time: 5 minutes

Cooking Time: 6 minutes

Servings: 1

Ingredients:

- 1 cup grated cheddar cheese
- 2 eggs

Directions:

1. Preheat the waffle iron.
2. Beat the eggs, then add the grated cheddar cheese.
3. Make sure that the mixture is well combined.
4. Cook the mixture for about six minutes.

Nutrition:

- **Calories:** 460
- **Carbohydrates:** 2 g
- **Protein:** 44 g
- **Fat:** 33 g

Preparation Time: 45 minutes

Cooking Time: 15 minutes

Servings: 8

Ingredients:

- 3 eggs
- 1 ½ cups grated cheddar cheese

For Toppings:

- 4 Gala apples (1 ¼ lb.), chopped finely
- ½ tsp. ground cinnamon
- ¼ cup sugar
- 2 tbsp. butter, melted
- ¼ cup pecans, chopped
- ½ cup whipped cream

Directions:

1. Preheat the waffle iron.
2. Combine the eggs and cheese well.
3. Roughly 2 tbsp. is 1 mini chaffle.
4. Add the batter to the waffle iron and cook for about three minutes.
5. A total of eight chaffles can be made with this batter.
6. Allow to cool and start on the topping.

For Topping:

1. Take the butter and melt in the saucepan at medium heat.
2. Add the chopped apples and cook for two minutes, stirring often.
3. Add the cinnamon and sugar to the apples.
4. Mix the pecans into the mixture and stir in.
5. Cover the saucepan with a lid and cook for a further five minutes at a low temperature.
6. Apples should be cooked until tender.

Nutrition:

- **Calories:** 250
- **Carbohydrates:** 21 g
- **Protein:** 8 g
- **Fat:** 16 g

Preparation Time: 5 minutes

Cooking Time: 10 minutes

Servings: 2

Ingredients:

- 1 egg
- ½ cup grated mozzarella cheese
- 2 tbsp. almond flour, ALLERGY WARNING
- 1 tsp. vanilla extract
- 1 tsp. cinnamon
- 1 tsp. granulated sweetener choice

Directions:

1. Preheat your waffle iron.
2. Mix all the chaffle ingredients well.
3. Use half of the mixture and cook the chaffle for about five minutes.
4. Add an extra minute to the cooking if you want a crispier chaffle.
5. Repeat until all the batter is used.

Nutrition:

- **Calories:** 180
- **Carbohydrates:** 7 g
- **Protein:** 11 g
- **Fat:** 12 g

295. Banana Nut Chaffle

Preparation Time: 3 minutes

Cooking Time: 8 minutes

Servings: 2

Ingredients:

- 1 egg
- ¼ tsp. vanilla extract
- ¼ tsp. banana extract
- 1 tbsp. cream cheese, room temperature, and softened
- ½ cup grated mozzarella cheese
- 1 tbsp. monk fruit confectioners, or confectioners' sweetener choice
- 1 tbsp. sugar-free cheesecake pudding, optional

Toppings:

- Pecans
- Sugar-free caramel sauce. or keto-safe sauce preference

Directions:

1. Preheat the waffle iron.
2. Beat the egg before adding the other ingredients, and make sure that everything is coated in the egg mixture.
3. Use half of the batter and cook for about four minutes.
4. Remove chaffle to rest while cooking the second mini chaffle.

Nutrition:

- **Calories:** 119
- **Carbohydrates:** 2.7 g
- **Protein:** 8.8 g
- **Fat:** 7.8 g

Preparation Time: 5 minutes

Cooking Time: 20 minutes

Servings: 4

Ingredients:

- 4 large eggs
- 1 cup almond flour, ALLERGY WARNING
- 1/3 cup flaxseed meal
- 1 tsp. vanilla extract
- ½ medium banana, slightly overripe
- 4 oz. cream cheese
- 2 tsp. baking powder
- ½ tsp. banana extract, optional
- Liquid stevia or sweetener choice, optional

For Banana Foster Topping:

- 8 tbsp. salted butter
- ½ tsp. cinnamon
- ½ tsp. vanilla extract
- ½ tsp. banana extract
- ¼ cup sugar-free maple syrup
- ½ cup brown sugar substitute or granulated sweetener with maple extract
- ½ medium banana, sliced into discs
- ¼ tsp. xanthan gum, optional
- 2 tbsp. dark rum or bourbon, optional
- ¼ cup pecans chopped, optional

Directions:

1. Preheat the waffle iron or skillet.
2. Add all the chaffle ingredients to a blender and blend until smooth.
3. Add ¼ of the batter to the waffle iron and cook for about two-three minutes; add an extra minute to cooking if the chaffle isn't set.

4. Repeat until all the batter is used.

Topping:

1. At a medium temperature, combine the banana extract, rum or bourbon, butter, and vanilla in a skillet.
2. As the mixture starts to bubble, add the sliced bananas in a single layer and allow them to cook for between two to three minutes. Do not stir.
3. After the time has passed, add the cinnamon, brown sugar substitute, and sugar-free maple syrup.
4. Stir and let the mixture simmer until all the brown sugar substitute has become melted and incorporated into the butter.
5. If the brown sugar substitute isn't blending with the butter, add the xanthan gum to the mixture. This will also help to thicken up the sauce.
6. Depending on your preference, you can either add the pecans to the simmering sauce or add it after pouring the source on the chaffles.
7. Add the warm sauce to the cooled chaffles.
8. Add a scoop or two of keto-friendly ice cream to make a unique taste experience. Or simply enjoy the chaffle with no sauce.

Nutrition:

- **Calories**: 417
- **Carbohydrates**: 13 g
- **Protein**: 10 g
- **Fat**: 37 g

Preparation Time: 3 minutes

Cooking Time: 8 minutes

Servings: 2

Ingredients:

- ½ cup grated mozzarella cheese
- ½ tbsp. granulated Swerve, or sweetener choice
- 1 tbsp. almond flour, ALLERGY WARNING
- 2 tbsp. low carb, sugar-free chocolate chips
- 1 egg
- ¼ tsp. cinnamon

Directions:

1. Preheat your waffle iron.
2. In a bowl, mix the almond flour, egg, cinnamon, mozzarella cheese, Swerve, chocolate chips.
3. Place half the batter in the waffle iron and cook for four minutes.
4. Remove chaffle and cook the remaining batter.
5. Let chaffles cool before serving.
6. Enjoy these chaffles with some keto-safe chocolate sauce and some whipped cream.

Nutrition:

- **Calories:** 136
- **Carbohydrates:** 2 g
- **Protein:** 10 g
- **Fat:** 10 g

Preparation Time: 3 minutes

Cooking Time: 5 minutes

Servings: 1

Ingredients:

- 1 tsp. vanilla extract
- 1 tbsp. cocoa powder, unsweetened.
- 1 egg
- 2 tbsp. almond flour, ALLERGY WARNING
- 2 tsp. monk fruit
- 1 oz. cream cheese

Directions:

1. Preheat the waffle iron.
2. Soften the cream cheese, then whisk together the other ingredients well.
3. Pour the batter into the center of the waffle iron and spread out.
4. Cook batter for between three and five minutes.
5. Remove chaffle once set and serve.
6. Consider making your own keto-friendly ice cream to go with this treatment so that you can enjoy it while it is still warm.

Nutrition:

- **Calories:** 261
- **Carbohydrates:** 4 g
- **Protein:** 11.5 g
- **Fat:** 22.2 g

Preparation Time: 30 minutes

Cooking Time: 20 minutes

Servings: 1

Ingredients:

- 1 egg
- ½ tsp. vanilla extract
- ¼ cup cream cheese
- 2 tsp. almond flour, ALLERGY WARNING
- 1 tbsp. sweetener choice
- 1 tbsp. protein powder, unflavored
- ½ tsp. baking powder
- 1 tsp. ground cinnamon

For Sugar-Free Marshmallow:

- 100 g (3.5 oz.) xylitol, or other baking friendly sweetener
- 3 tbsp. water
- 4 gelatin sheets, or 7 g gelatin powder

For Chocolate Dip:

- 10 g cacao butter
- 80 g sugar-free chocolate

Directions:

For Sugar-Free Marshmallow:

1. If you do not have sugar-free marshmallow fluff, then it is suggested that you make this up to eight hours, or even the day before, making the chaffle.
2. Choose a container to set the marshmallow in later. This container needs to be lined with cling film.
3. Gelatin sheets need to be placed in water for a few minutes before use.
4. Melt the sugar in a cooking pot and allow to boil for up to three minutes before adding the gelatin sheets or powder.
5. Dissolve the gelatin fully.
6. Now that the liquid is ready, pour it into an electric mixer.

7. Mix the mixture until the liquid bulks up and starts to form a white marshmallow-like fluff.
8. Pour the marshmallow fluff into the earlier prepared container and smooth the surface.
9. Allow the mixture to sit on a kitchen surface for no less than eight hours. For the best possible setting, allow the fluff to rest overnight to set into the marshmallow form. Cover with cling film once cool to prevent insects from getting into the mixture.
10. Once fully set, the marshmallow can be cut into the desired shape.
11. Dust the marshmallow pieces with powdered sweetener if you want to keep it softer for longer.

Chaffle:

1. Preheat the waffle iron.
2. Beat the egg before adding the cinnamon.
3. Combine the remaining chaffle ingredients before adding a few drops of vanilla.
4. Divide the batter in half and cook each portion for three minutes.
5. Set chaffles aside to cool.
6. If you want to prepare the S'mores at home, take the marshmallow fluff and spread it to the thickness of choice on one chaffle before adding the second chaffle on top.
7. Set aside the chaffles to prepare the chocolate dip.

For Chocolate Dip:

1. Make use of a double boiler or instant pot to melt the cocoa butter and sugar-free chocolate together.
2. Make sure the mixture is completely smooth before dipping the chaffles edges in it. Coat all the marshmallow fluff.
3. Put aside and allow the chocolate to harden.
4. Whether you are making this as a snack at home or you take the individual parts with you to go camping, this chaffle is something that is a must in your collection.

Nutrition:

- **Calories**: 368
- **Carbohydrates**: 3 g
- **Protein**: 11 g
- **Fat**: 23 g

300. Thin Mint Cookie Chaffles

Preparation Time: 20 minutes

Cooking Time: 16 minutes

Servings: 4

Ingredients:

- 1 cup grated mozzarella cheese
- 2 tbsp. unsweetened cocoa powder
- 2 large eggs
- 3 tbsp. Swerve confectioners or sweetener choice

For Filling:

- 6 oz. cream cheese, softened
- 2 tbsp. unsweetened cocoa powder
- ½ cup almond flour, ALLERGY WARNING
- ¼ cup Swerve confectioners, or sweeteners choice
- 1 tsp. peppermint extract
- ½ tsp. vanilla extract

For Topping:

- 3 tbsp. sugar-free chocolate chips
- 1 tbsp. coconut oil, ALLERGY WARNING

Directions:

1. Preheat the waffle iron.
2. Mix all the chaffle ingredients in a bowl and make sure everything is mixed well.
3. Cook ¼ of the batter in the waffle iron for two to four minutes. The longer it is cooked, the crispier it becomes.
4. Continue to make chaffles until the batter is finished.

For Filling and Topping:

5. Combine all the filler ingredients and beat with a hand mixer on high.
6. Apply the filling to the three cooled chaffles, stack, and set aside.

7. Heat the coconut oil and chocolate chips at 30-second intervals in a microwave until melted together.
8. Drizzle this over the stacked chaffles and serve.
9. Anyone who is a fan of chocolate will not turn their nose up at this treat!

Nutrition:

- **Calories**: 431
- **Carbohydrates**: 6 g
- **Protein**: 16 g
- **Fat**: 38 g

Chapter 10.

12 Tips for Making the Best Chaffles

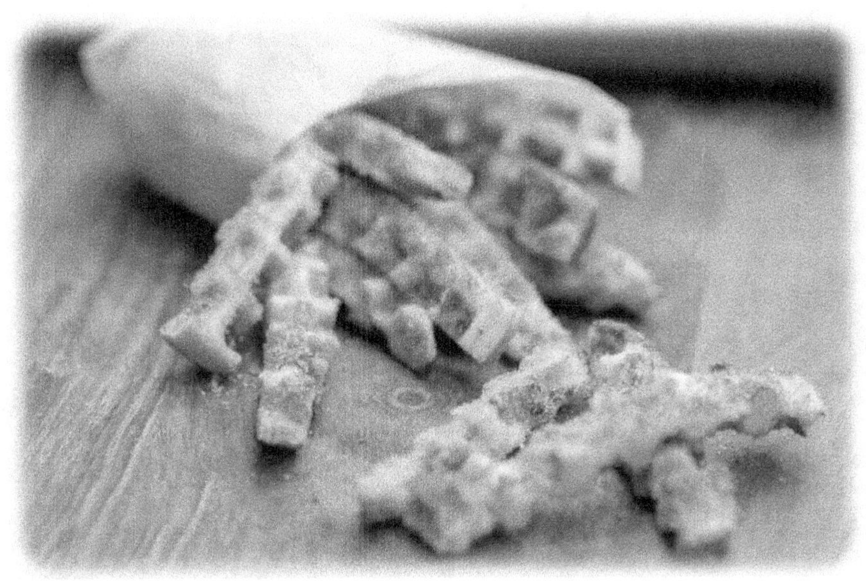

1. Use Full-fat Cheese

Always use full-fat cheese for making chaffles not only because it tastes better but because on a Keto diet, you should try to increase your fat intake whenever you can. Cheddar or mozzarella is the best, although you can also combine them at 50:50. You can also experiment with adding some cream cheese to shredded cheddar. Personally, I notice cream cheese gives a thick, softer consistency compared to mozzarella or cheddar

2. Add Ingredients Gradually

Start by placing a small handful of cheese in a small bowl, then add the egg, after which you can add the remaining cheese. When you add the ingredients gradually before pouring them into the waffle maker, the cheese will be distributed evenly, and you will get crispier chaffles.

3. Use a High-Heat Setting

You need a high-heat setting if you want to get crispy chaffles. Make sure your waffle maker is very hot before you add the chaffle batter. Always follow the manufacturer's instructions, but with the Dash mini waffle maker, the standard procedure is to plug it in and wait until the light goes off

4. Shred the Cheese Finely

Finely shredded cheese cooks well when it comes in thicker shreds. Besides, finely shredded cheese is more evenly distributed in the batter and ensures the chaffle is crisp all over rather than some parts being crispy while others remain soft and soggy.

5. Cook for at Least 3 Minutes

Mix the ingredients, spoon half the batter in a mini waffle maker, and cook for 3-5 minutes. When it's cooked, remove and repeat with the remaining batter. If you don't have a waffle maker but are cooking chaffles on an electric grid, you need to flip the chaffle after about 3-5 minutes and cook it for additional 3-5 minutes.

6. Let Chaffles Rest

After removing the cooked chaffle from the waffle maker, let it rest for a couple of minutes (on a cooling rack preferably) before serving it. However, don't let it stand for too long, for its best eaten warm.

7. To Get Chaffles with More Consistency

You can add some coconut flour or almond flour to give your chaffle a bread-like texture. It is not okay to use plain flour since your goal is to cut down on carbs as on the ketogenic diet. Adding flour to your chaffle recipe would not make this a Keto-friendly treat.

Serve it immediately. If possible, serve chaffles while they're still warm and top them with butter and sugar-free syrup, sugar-free jam, or a savory sauce of your choice.

8. To Make Your Chaffle Taste a Less Eggy

Instead of whole eggs, use two egg whites. This will slightly change the texture and the taste, but it won't taste eggy. Beat the egg whites until very firm, then gradually add the other ingredients.

9. Don't Open the Waffle Maker During the Cooking

Be patient and let the cheese form the crust, which it will not be able to do if you lift the cover to check if it's ready. If you interrupt the cooking process, the chaffle will be melty and sticky. Think about it in advance how long you want to cook it for (at least 3 minutes, but not more than 5) and let the cover of the waffle maker remain closed until fully done.

10. To Get a Crispy Crust

There are many tips on how to get a crisp crust, but the easiest one is to add 1 tsp. of shredded cheese to the preheated waffle maker of electric girdle before you add the batter. This will give a delicious crispy crust.

11. You Need the Right Heat

The waffle maker or the electric pan needs to be very hot before you add the batter, otherwise, the chaffle will not only not be crispy on the outside but will remain gooey on the inside. Depending on what appliances you are using, there are different ways of checking if the pan or waffle maker is hot enough.

12. Ensure Your Waffle Iron Has a Nice Non-stick Surface

Brush the waffle maker or electric pan with butter or oil, even if it's supposed to be a non-stick surface. I know many argue about the cheese in the batter being enough to prevent sticking but remember, old appliances tend to lose the non-stick quality, so the coating is necessary.

CONCLUSION

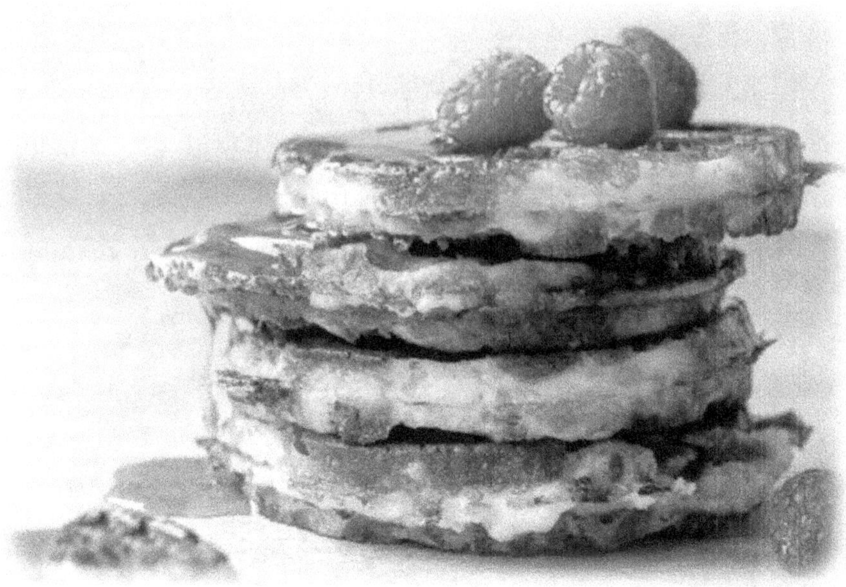

The Ketogenic diet believes that by minimizing your carbs, you will while maximizing the good fat in your system and making sure that you're getting the protein you need, that you will be happier and healthier Keto diet can be a complicated affair, especially when you are starting out, particularly when it comes to desserts, sugary food, and some diary stuff. If you are an ardent keto diet follower, low-carb chaffles are super-easy to make, and the ingredients are readily accessible in your local supermarket or grocery store.

Regularly, keto dieters look out for ways to be accurate on the diet while searching for ways to make life easier at that. Chaffles are one of those foods that bring on a stimulating effect to the low-carb lifestyle. Now, there isn't the need to deal with bulky, flour-stuffed pastries when cheese and egg offer a better version. This blend, therefore, makes dieting simpler as chaffles are enriched with healthy fat and mostly with no carbs.

Reaching ketosis just got easier!

Finally, they are convenient for prep-ahead meals. And we know how prepping meals aids with effective keto dieting. Chaffles can be frozen for later use, and they taste excellent when warmed and enjoyed later.

414

Once you are hooked on chaffles, they will become a crucial part of your feeding because of their benefits. As soon as you quickly fall in love with chaffles, you will find that there are two major ways to enjoy them: sweet and savory. With that said, just like any other food, the key to making your chaffles tasty is by having the right tools and owning the ingredients.

Here are some of my tips that will help you to make incredibly tasty chaffle recipes.

Many, if not all, chaffle recipes require you to use a tablespoon of baking powder or almond flour to give them a slightly more waffle-like texture and make them crispier.

Another tip for preparing really tasty chaffles is giving them ample time to cook. Always avoid opening the waffle prematurely, as it may affect the doneness or crispness of your chaffles. If anything, the best chaffles tend to be those that are cooked for a slightly longer period.

From time to time, the phenomenon of food breaks open and unexpected worlds, burning social media like wildfires and sweeping out innocents like tsunamis. What is this natural force?

This is the case for chaffle. The waffle is made entirely of cheese and eggs. Sprinkle the minced cheese directly on a hot waffle iron, add some of the beaten eggs, put the cheese on top, and leave it to the waffle maker.

For people who are on the go and have a busy lifestyle, we have provided easy recipes so that you can make food quickly and have a great meal for your lifestyle. It also has enough servings for leftovers in the morning on the next day to pack it up and take it with you wherever you go. This works out so much easier for so many people because they don't have to cook in the morning, and it saves a busy person a lot of time.

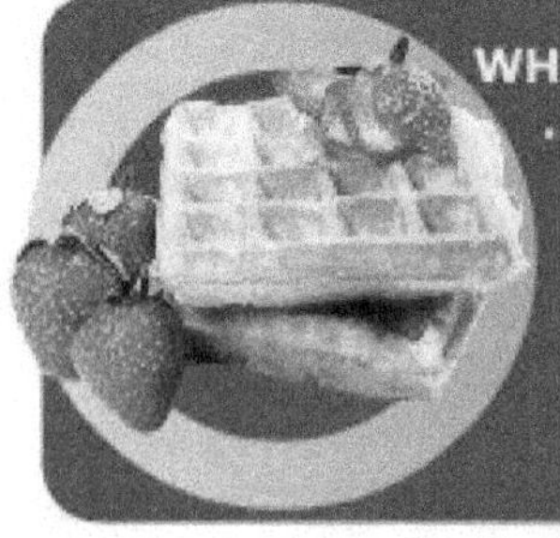

WHAT IS A CHAFFLE?

no one really knows who first coined the term

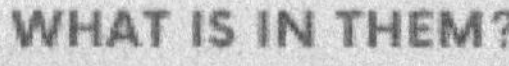

WHAT IS IN THEM?

chaffles are just waffles and yummy cheese

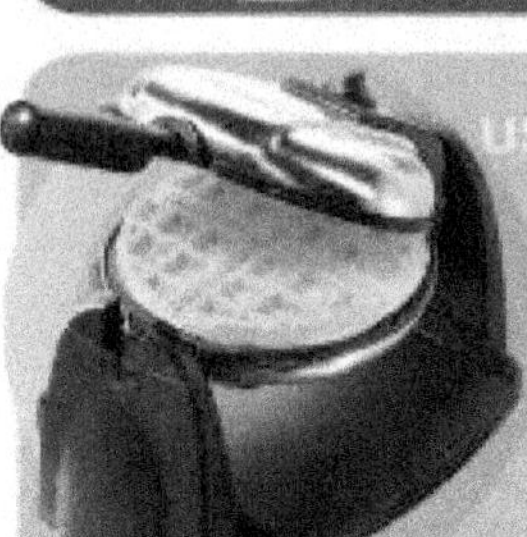

USE A WAFFLE IRON

a waffle iron is ideal for cooking delicious chaffles

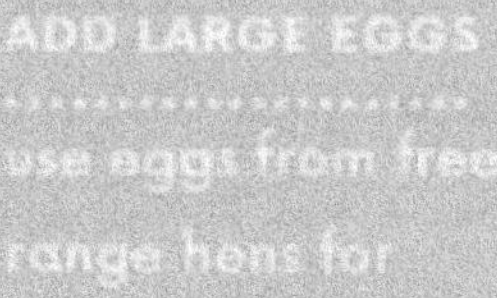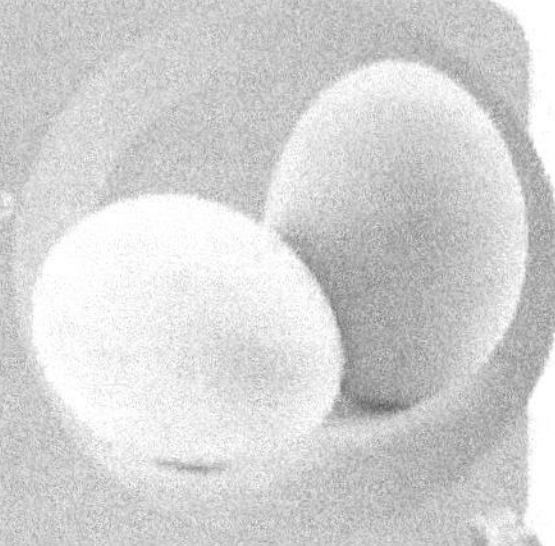

ADD LARGE EGGS

use eggs from free range hens for extra consistency

ADD FRESH BERRIES

garnish your chaffles with healthy berries

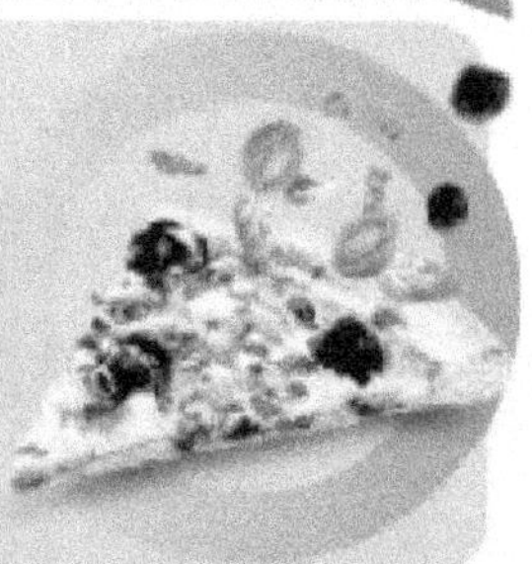

SO MANY RECIPES

try pizza flavored chaffles, or even pumpkin perhaps

YUMMY TOPPINGS

add lush syrups and toppings for extra flavor

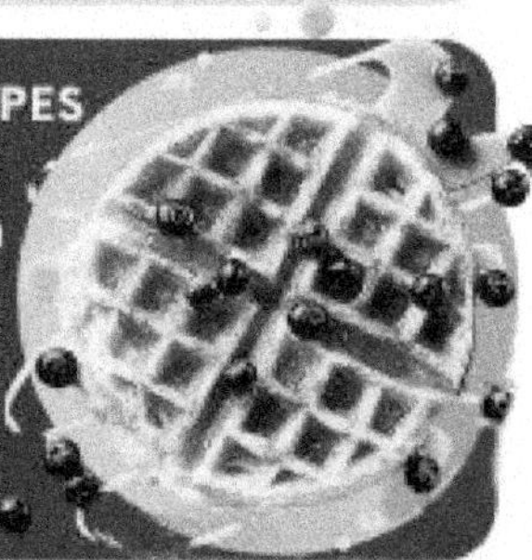

10+ CHAFFLE RECIPES

keep it sweet with more keto chaffle recipe ideas...